The Vaccination Dilemma

"The Vaccination Dilemma gives parents more than pros and cons about childhood vaccinations. It reveals an alternative health care system that removes much of the fear from childhood disease. This book suggests parents grow beyond the "one size fits all" system of health care and understand that every illness serves a unique need for every unique child, and that health enhancement rather than disease treatment is the future of modern health care."

—**Tedd Koren, D.C.**, author, *Childhood Vaccination:*
Questions Every Parent Should Ask

"A fine book . . . the powerful philosophies of anthroposophy and homeopathy provide unique perspectives that can help parents to trust themselves and their children's innate wisdom."

—**Peggy O'Mara**, editor and publisher, *Mothering Magazine*

"This book illuminates for the reader, as no other book to my knowledge has done, the underlying reality of our immune mechanisms in regard to acute inflammatory diseases, our response to them, and the still questionable value of purposeful immunizations. This book should be read by all physicians, health care providers, and families with children."

—**John R. Lee, M.D.**

The Vaccination Dilemma

Christine Murphy, Editor

Lantern Books ● New York
A Division of Booklight Inc

2002
Lantern Books
One Union Square West, Suite 201
New York, NY 10003

None of the material in this book is meant to replace the advice of
your physician.

Cover photograph by Amy K. Pickering

Printed in the United States of America

Library of Congress Cataloging-in-Publication Data　.

The Vaccination Dilemma / Christine Murphy, editor
    p. cm.
Includes bibliographical references.
  ISBN 1-930051-10-7
  1. Vaccination of children. 2. Anthroposophical therapy. I. Murphy,
Christine.
RJ240 .V324 2002
614.47'083—dc21

2002007898

Inflammation is a reaction, a healing mechanism aimed at eliminating foreign substances or processes, and we must know how to respect it. It would be a grave error to combat it in all circumstances. It may happen that it constitutes in itself a danger through its intensity or localization, and in that case it is the duty of the doctor to moderate it, but to dispel it without due consideration would be to risk being shipwrecked by Scylla while avoiding Charybdis, and would expose the organism to no less a danger, albeit possibly at a later date.

—**Victor Bott, M.D.**, from *Spiritual Science and the Art of Healing*, Healing Arts Press, Vermont, 1996

✎ Acknowledgments

M any of the following offerings are reprints of articles that have appeared in the complementary health quarterly *Lilipoh*. Others were written especially for this collection. We are grateful for the writers' wisdom and experience, which translate into insights and help for the reader.

Special thanks to Barbara Loe Fisher for her ongoing research, to Philip Incao, M.D., who contributed three important articles and oversaw the medical editing, to Sarah Gallogly of Lantern Books for her suggestions and editing, and to the providers in the resource section for their dedication to child health and well-being.

❦ Contents

✌ Foreword

Wiep de Vries, R.N.

The news is out: vaccination is not as safe as some would have us believe. Worried parents have taken the initiative and started learning about the possible links between chronic illness and vaccinations. While there is no doubt that vaccines can be a blessing in times of real danger, concerned parents are now leading the way to wake us up to a critical issue: vaccines may leave children with permanent damage or severe chronic illness. Numerous organizations are networking worldwide to disseminate studies and personal stories that alert others to the potential toxicity of vaccinations as an assault on the immune system, especially in the very first years of life.

Some parents carefully select the vaccines they feel most comfortable with. Developing immunity the old-fashioned way is also becoming popular. I regularly get calls from parents wanting to expose their children to chicken pox, asking whether I know any kids who have it. More and more parents opt out of the many vaccines every child is supposed to have before going to school, as the news spreads about links between vaccines and autism (a 273% increase in autism in California over the last ten years), seizures, asthma, arthritis, Crohn's disease, and even hyperactivity and learning disabilities.

As a nurse and health educator, I have watched many parents struggle emotionally with concerns about the known risks of vaccines and of the illnesses they were invented to fight. As they increase their knowledge, they come to question more deeply what lies behind their fear of illness. "Take your time to decide," I always advise. The life and health of a child are too precious to compromise.

We have lost the connection to practical folk wisdom, once transmitted by our mothers and grandmothers. Most parents feel quite lost, especially in the midst of all the media messages about the frightening effects of illnesses.

Be informed and stay connected with your inner voice of wisdom. Ask yourself: "What is it that I need in order to address my fears? Is it the knowledge and reassurance of a trustworthy health practitioner who will stand behind me? How can I build trust in my capability to take care of my child?"

I see it as the ultimate act of courage when parents take full responsibility for the vaccination decision, taking time to discuss their options and to study the potential risks of each. Don't hold back asking crucial questions, and prepare the ground for a support network, including a doctor, to help you cope in times of illness. With careful research, no matter what conclusions you draw, you will become better able to keep your children safe.

> **Remember:**
> - Every child is an individual and needs individual evaluation.
> - Travel to other countries imposes a new set of rules.
> - An epidemic and an isolated occurrence require different responses.
> - Find a physician you can trust and work with.

➣ Introduction

Christine Murphy

Anyone who has held a feverish infant knows the anxious question: am I providing the right care? We may well believe that childhood illnesses have spiritual significance, yet our courage may fail us at the thought of them. Vaccination seems to be the answer to our anxiety, yet controversy is growing over its wise and appropriate use.

This book wishes to create a basis for informed decisions regarding vaccinations, explaining when children are most vulnerable and what can be done to minimize possible side effects. With the exception of the opening report by Barbara Loe Fisher of the National Vaccine Information Center, the book's contributors are practitioners representing a unique view of illness, based in the traditions of homeopathic and anthroposophical medicine. The latter, inaugurated by Rudolf Steiner in 1920 and developed since then by physicians, nurses, and therapists in Europe and around the world, states that illness is rarely a random or accidental event. It is usually a purposeful transformational process in the life of an individual child or adult. Healing takes place through those measures that support and facilitate the safe completion of this transformational process.

Vaccines are just one factor in a young child's health, and most vaccinated children do just fine in later life. But a disturbing and growing body of research implies that indiscriminate prevention may result in shifting the physical expression of children's illnesses from acute to chronic diseases. Another concern is that vaccinations and other suppressive treatments may thwart much-needed inflammatory remodeling and transformation, affecting the healthy growth of the child's spirit in the realm of consciousness, emotions, and neurological maturity. This could account for today's disturbing incidence of behavioral, psychological, and neurological problems in our children.

Are we practicing "insurance," hoping to avoid all unpleasantness that might befall our children? Do we realize what the cost of this may be? Modern science must accurately assess this cost so that health policy and parental decision can be guided by objective facts.

Parents are becoming aware that the childhood illnesses that claim so many young lives in developing countries today pose relatively little risk in modern societies. Out of their years of experience and generations of children seen through to a healthy adulthood, our authors offer an overview of some common childhood illnesses and information on how to treat them, how to prepare your child for vaccination, how to find support for whatever road you choose, and how to cope with illness without undue fear.

In truth, we are all caregivers—whether or not we feel we have chosen that office—and the more informed we become, the better we'll care for our loved ones.

Part I

The Problem with Vaccination

National Vaccine Information Center Report

Barbara Loe Fisher

As guardians of their children until those children are old enough to make life-and-death decisions for themselves, parents take very seriously the responsibility of making informed vaccination decisions for the children they love. However, relatively few parents are aware of the risks of injury that some vaccines can present. This article will help educate parents about these risks and prepare them to make, in consultation with one or more health professionals, an educated vaccination decision for their child.

Like every encounter with a viral or bacterial infection, every vaccine containing lab-altered viruses or bacteria has an inherent ability to cause injury. Vaccination can either produce immunity without incident or result in mild to severe brain and immune system damage, depending upon the vaccine or combination of vaccines given, the health of the person at the time of vaccination, and whether the individual is genetically or otherwise biologically at risk for developing complications.

The fact that vaccines can cause injury and death was officially acknowledged in the U.S. in 1986, when Congress passed the National Childhood Vaccine Injury Act, creating a no-fault federal compensation system for vaccine-injured children to protect vaccine manufacturers and doctors from vaccine injury lawsuits. Since then, the system has paid out nearly $1.3 billion to families whose loved ones have died or been harmed by vaccines.

Since 1990, between 12,000 and 14,000 reports of hospitalizations, injuries, and deaths following vaccination have been made to the federal Vaccine Adverse Event Reporting System (VAERS) annually, but it is estimated that only between one and ten percent of all doctors make reports to VAERS. Therefore, the number of vaccine-related health problems occurring in the U.S. every year may well number over one million.

In the late 1980s, the Institute of Medicine (IOM)-National Academy of Sciences convened committees of physicians to study existing medical knowledge about vaccines. In 1991 and 1994, IOM issued historic reports confirming that vaccines can cause death and a wide spectrum of brain and immune system damage. But the most important conclusion, which deserves greater public attention and congressional action, was that "[t]he lack of adequate data regarding many of the [vaccine] adverse events under study was of major concern to the committee ... the committee encountered many gaps and limitations in knowledge bearing directly or indirectly on the safety of vaccines."

Because so little medical research has been conducted into vaccine side effects, no tests have been developed to identify and screen out vulnerable children. As a result, public health officials have taken a "one-size-fits-all" approach and have aggressively implemented mandatory vaccination laws while dismissing children who are injured or die after vaccination as unfortunate but necessary sacrifices "for the greater good." This utilitarian rationale is of little comfort to the growing numbers of mothers and fathers who vaccinate their healthy, bright children, then watch them die suddenly or develop mental retardation, epilepsy, learning and behavior disorders, autism, diabetes, arthritis, or asthma.

As vaccination rates have approached ninety-eight percent for children entering kindergarten in many states, there is no question that mass vaccination in the past quarter century has suppressed infectious diseases in childhood, lowering the incidence of measles in the western hemisphere from a high of over 400,000 cases in 1965 to only 100 in 1999. Yet, even as infectious disease rates have fallen, rates of chronic disease and disability among children and young adults have risen dramatically.

A University of California study published by the U.S. Department of Education in 1996 found that "the proportion of the U.S. population with disabilities has risen markedly during the past quarter century . . . this recent change seems to be due not to demographics, but to greater numbers of children and young adults reported as having disabilities." The study concluded that the change was due to "increases in the prevalence of asthma, mental disorders (including attention deficit disorder), mental retardation and learning disabilities that have been noted among children in recent years."

Instead of epidemics of measles, we have epidemics of chronic autoimmune and neurological disease: in the past twenty-five years, rates of asthma and attention deficit disorder have doubled; diabetes and learning disabilities have tripled; chronic arthritis now affects nearly one in five Americans; and autism has increased by 300 percent or more in many states. The larger, unanswered question is: To what extent has the administration of multiple doses of multiple vaccines in early childhood—when the body's brain and immune system are developing at their most rapid rate—been a co-factor in epidemics of chronic disease? The assumption that mass vaccination policies have played no role is as unscientific and dangerous as the assumption that an individual child's health problems following vaccination are only coincidentally related to the vaccination.

Outstanding questions about vaccination can only be answered by basic science research into the biological mechanism of vaccine injury and death so that pathological profiles can be developed to distinguish between vaccine-induced and unrelated health problems. Whether the gaps in scientific knowledge about vaccines will be filled in this decade or remain unanswered in the next depends upon the funding and research priorities set by Congress, the National Institutes of Health (NIH), and industry.

With the understanding that medical science and the doctors who practice it are not infallible, today's better-educated health care consumer is demanding more information, more choices, and a more equal decision-making partnership with doctors. Young parents, who are being told that their children must be injected with thirty-seven doses of eleven different vaccines before the age of five, are asking questions, like: Why does my newborn infant have to be injected with hepatitis B vaccine when I am not infected with hepatitis B and my infant is not an IV drug user or engaging in sex with multiple partners—the two highest risk groups for hepatitis B infection? And: Why does my twelve-month-old have to get chicken pox vaccine when chicken pox is a mild disease and once my child gets it, he or she will be immune for life?

Informed parents know that hepatitis B is not like polio, and chicken pox is not like smallpox. They know the difference between taking a risk with a vaccine for an adult disease that is hard to catch, like the blood-transmitted hepatitis B, and using a vaccine to prevent a devastating, highly contagious childhood disease like polio. All diseases and all vaccines are not the same, and neither are children.

Parents understand the qualitative difference between options freely taken and punishing dictates. They are calling for enlightened, humane implementation of state vaccination laws, including insertion of informed consent protections that strengthen exemptions for sincerely held religious or conscientious beliefs. This is especially critical for parents with reason to believe that their child may be at high risk of injury or death from one or more vaccines, who cannot find a doctor to write a medical exemption.

Informed consent has been the gold standard in the ethical practice of medicine since World War II, acknowledging the human right of individuals or their guardians to make fully informed, voluntary decisions about whether to undergo a medical procedure that could result in harm or death. To the extent that vaccination has been exempted from informed consent protections, and vaccine makers and doctors have been exempted from liability for vaccine injuries and deaths, the notion that a minority of individuals are expendable in service to the majority has prevented a real commitment of will and resources to develop ways to screen vulnerable children out and spare their lives. It is not difficult to understand why some parents resist offering up their children as sacrifices for a policy they believe lacks scientific and moral integrity.

But even as educated health care consumers are asking for more information and choices, mechanisms are being set up to restrict those choices. Government-operated electronic vaccine tracking systems are already in place in most states, using health care identifier numbers to tag and track children without the parents' informed consent in order to enforce use of all government-recommended vaccines now and in the future. HMOs are turning down children for health insurance, and federal entitlement programs are economically punishing parents who cannot show proof that their child got every state-recommended vaccine. Even children who have suffered severe vaccine reactions are being pressured to get re-vaccinated or be barred from getting an education.

Drug companies and federal agencies are developing more than two hundred new vaccines, including ones for gonorrhea and herpes that will target twelve-year olds. On March 2, 2000, President Clinton joined with the international pharmaceutical industry, multinational banks, and the Bill and Melinda Gates Foundation to launch the Millennium Vaccine Initiative, committing several billion dollars to vaccinating all children in the world with existing and future vaccines, including those in accelerated development for AIDS, TB, and malaria. Since the terrifying events of September 11, 2001, which were followed by threats of biological warfare in cities across America, there have been calls for inoculation of all American children and adults with anthrax and smallpox vaccines. In any mass vaccination campaign there will be casualties and, if history repeats itself, both industry and government will be reluctant to take steps to minimize those casualties or to admit that they occur.

With so many unanswered questions about vaccine safety, but with the knowledge that every vaccine carries an inherent risk and that some individuals will be more vulnerable to vaccine reactions than others, the right to informed consent to vaccination takes on even greater legal and ethical significance as we head into the twenty-first century. In a broader sense, the concept of informed consent transcends medicine and addresses the constitutional concept of civil liberty, the ethical concept of individual inviolability, and the right to self-determination. Forced vaccination policies, which are implemented by public health officials through state vaccine mandates, too often take a "no exceptions" stance. The question now becomes: If the state can tag, track down, and force individuals against their will to be injected with biologicals of unknown toxicity today, will there be any limit on what individual freedoms the state can take away in the name of the greater good tomorrow?

Parents, who know and love their children better than anyone else, have the human right to make informed, voluntary vaccination decisions for their children without facing state-sanctioned punishment. Whether a child is hurt by a vaccine or a disease, it is the mother and father—not the pediatrician, vaccine maker, or public health official—who will bear the lifelong grief and burden of what happens to that child.

❦ An Anthroposophical Perspective

Robert Zieve, M.D.

V accinations have today become part of the accepted protocol in raising children. They are in the same almost universally accepted category as fever suppressants, antibiotics, milk, and apple pie (and refined carbohydrates in general). However, the accumulation of these assaults on a child's constitution have had harmful effects. This article will more specifically discuss the impact of vaccines on the growth and development of the child.

The principle behind vaccinations is to prevent disease. The idea is that if a child does not contract measles, or chicken pox, or other contagious diseases, then he or she will have a better chance of living a healthy life. From an anthroposophical perspective, we know that when we permit the child to go through one of these childhood illnesses, receiving treatment with natural remedies that greatly minimize the occurrence of complications, he or she emerges from this illness stronger. More specifically, the immune system is stronger. Many people have observed how after one of these illnesses the child's constitution and emerging temperament change for the better.

It is often claimed that vaccinations are the reason we do not have epidemics anymore. The reality is that many of the infectious diseases against which children are being immunized were declining dramatically in Western nations before the introduction of immunizations. This was due to improvements in social hygiene, and to other factors related to modernization. For example, there was a 99.8% decline in tetanus in the military between the Civil War and World War II, before tetanus immunizations were introduced. In 1978, the magazine *Science* estimated that forty percent of the population was not protected against tetanus, yet the incidence of the disease declined. Epidemics of infectious diseases are connected to human relations with each other and with the earth, and vaccinations address neither of these relationships.

What is our role in helping a child grow and develop? Each person has a destiny that he or she will meet, in stages, during life. Is it not our role to do our best to prepare this child to be strong enough to recognize, meet, and engage these forces of destiny? If it is, then part of this role is to help children overcome any forces that stand as obstacles on this path, without doing the work for them. When children develop one of these contagious diseases, this represents the efforts of their constitution to overcome latent blockages that, if not overcome early, may pose problems later.

Behind the immunization policy today is a view that all illness is bad and to be avoided and prevented. The issue of immunizations often is clouded by fear, as the mental clarity of perception is clouded by fears of death.[1] Too often today, science rules by fear. Until we change our collective approach from one of fearing illness to one of meeting illness as an integral part of a transformative life, we will create a lot of unnecessary problems for many children.

* * *

What are some of the problems we see as a result of the current immunization proliferation? They can include outbreaks of measles and other childhood contagious diseases in adolescence and young adulthood, at a time of life when they can cause far more complications than in early life. Our compulsion to vaccinate has also contributed significantly to the epidemic of autism in children. In addition, the growing incidence of chronic neurodegenerative illnesses and cancer later in life are increasingly thought to have a hidden viral component. Viruses stored inside cells become RNA and DNA hybrids that change cellular dynamics. We know that a major problem today is premature sclerosis, or hardening, of the nervous system and other organs.

In fact, with our national immunization policy, we have made a trade. We think that with immunizations we have decreased the incidence of many contagious diseases of childhood. It is likely that a few deaths from measles encephalitis and whooping cough have been prevented. But in return, have we contributed to the development of autism in children, and of chronic incapacitating illnesses in thousands of adults? What is the relationship between these disorders and vaccinations?

In autism, and autistic spectrum disorders, children suddenly begin to withdraw from the incarnational process. They stop making eye contact, repeat for weeks phrases heard on television, become oversensitive to sense stimuli. They become deficient in what has been called social intelligence. These and other signs and symptoms all point to a withdrawal of the "I," the individualizing ego, and a regression into repetition. These children will not recover without significant dietary restrictions. Their nervous systems become toxic with long-chain fatty acids.

There is increasing evidence that vaccinations have played an important role in the epidemic of autism. More specifically, the measles, mumps, and rubella (MMR) and hepatitis B vaccines have been the two most implicated. These change the entire milieu of the intestines, leading to the breakdown of a healthy self/not-self barrier. As a consequence, wild peptides are generated in the gut and absorbed into the nervous system, where they often become toxic. When present in large enough amounts in the autistic child, they can distort thinking and perceptions and lead to hallucinations or overstimulation.

People with Crohn's disease, a chronic inflammation of the small intestine that occurs in teens and young adults, have been found to have measles virus in the mucosa of the small intestine much more often if they have received immunizations as a child. The introduction of routine measles immunization with live measles virus coincided with a marked increase in Crohn's in the United Kingdom. A study in the medical journal *Lancet* revealed that a person is three times as likely to develop Crohn's if he or she has received the measles vaccine.

The role of heavy metal accumulation, especially mercury, from cumulative doses of thimerosol in almost all vaccinations, is also important. Mercury alters our immune response to foods and damages intestinal permeability, so it affects our ability to mediate self and not-self. This ability is severely impaired in autistic children.

The immune system is an organ of our "I." It registers the memory of prior exposures in order to protect the integrity of our life. Immunizations exhaust the immune capacity. A large number of T-lymphocytes become involved with antigens (specific protein particles) of the vaccines, and so are unavailable for other work in our differentiation of self and not-self. Furthermore, the foreign protein/live virus of the vaccine goes directly into the body without having to go through the liver like other protein. This bypasses the body's self-recognition capacities.

The result of the cumulative distortions of the terrain by immunizations, sugars, antibiotics, hormones, over-intellectualized education, and other commonly accepted approaches with children is an increasing number of children and adults whose souls and spiritual natures have difficulty living in their physical bodies.

In essence, what we are doing on a societal level is preventing, on a large scale, the growth and development of healthy adults with a strong "I," who are prepared to meet and fulfill their destiny, in order to allegedly save a few children from dying from these infectious diseases. The veracity of even this is questionable, because it is well documented that during major flu and other infectious epidemics earlier in the last century, the incidence of deaths in children who were treated homeopathically was much lower than in the general population.

* * *

If parents intend not to immunize, it is essential that they do this in collaboration with a professional or other individuals who are trained in the anthroposophical, homeopathic, or other traditional approaches to caring for children so that they are not overwhelmed by the consequences of the illness, but can go through it and emerge stronger. It is also essential that parents familiarize themselves with the signs and symptoms of the illnesses that are immunized against, so that they may work consciously and actively with trained professionals in guiding their children to greater states of health.

Today, humankind is collectively going through what the psychologist Dr. Bernard Lievegoed has called a "threshold experience." This means that we are in the process of taking a big leap forward in consciousness that challenges us to a deeper expression of our dormant capacities, feelings, and awareness. We see this in the widespread interest in the afterlife, in the many people who seek avenues of self-transformation, and in efforts to change the cultural, political, and economic spheres of human interaction. Yet there is little real freedom of thinking today when it comes to immunizations. If our goal is to ensure healthy children, then we must recognize the necessity of childhood disease in the developmental process, learn how to protect and guide our children through these illnesses, and develop clear thinking with respect to immunizations, building a decision process that is free of fear and coercion. Acute illness in childhood, if guided correctly, prevents chronic disease at a later time in life, and permits a deeper uniting of body, soul, and spirit as a unified whole. This allows the emergence of human goodness and creativity, benefiting our entire society.

1. Robert Sardello addresses this in his excellent book *Freeing the Soul from Fear* (Riverhead Books, 1999).

Reflections on Immunity, Vaccination, and Smallpox

Philip Incao, M.D.

Part One: The Phenomenon of Immunity

Illness is a process that all people experience repeatedly in their lifetime. Until our modern era, illnesses were classified according to their recognizable signs and symptoms. Today, we also classify them according to unique features detectable with the microscope and biochemical tests. Thus many illnesses of similar or identical appearance that were lumped together in the past can now be distinguished from one another based on their microscopic or biochemical features. For example, what for hundreds of years was called influenza is now described as a group of "influenza-like illnesses," each one associated with a different virus.

On the other hand, many diseases known for centuries and recognizable by their typical signs and symptoms have been confirmed by modern science to be distinct entities—that is, each is associated with its own particular virus or bacterium and with no other. Measles, chicken pox, and scarlet fever are examples of these. It has long been known that in such illnesses, one experience of the illness usually confers lifelong immunity. A second experience with measles or scarlet fever is extremely rare.

These observations by physicians and patients throughout history, in addition to careful observations of the stages in a patient's recovery from an acute inflammatory illness like measles or scarlet fever, have led to certain basic concepts in medicine.

One of these concepts was formulated as "Hering's Law" in the nineteenth century, although it was well-recognized and mentioned by the ancient Greek physician Hippocrates. This law states that as an illness resolves, its manifest signs and symptoms travel from the inner vital organs and blood circulation to the outer surface of the body, often visible as a rash or as a discharge of blood, mucus, or pus. In this way we "throw off" an illness.

Another basic concept arising from the phenomenology of illness, i.e., from observations of the directly perceptible behavior of human illness, is the concept of immunity to or protection from an illness that one has had before. This immunity to second episodes of certain illnesses, like measles or scarlet fever, reveals a *knowing* function of the human body in relation to illness. This inner knowing allows us, without any conscious knowledge or effort, to recognize an illness we've had before and to thereby resist it or quickly repulse it. Hering's law, on the other hand, is evidence of an innate *doing* function in healing: we actively clear the illness from our body; we get it out of our system as we heal.

These inner activities of doing and knowing, which work more strongly during illness than in the healthy state, were clearly recognized by the ancient physicians. Hippocrates said illness consisted of the active element *pónos* (labor) as well as the passive element *pathos* (suffering). Illness is intense inner work. Hippocrates perceived this labor as a cooking and digesting (*pepsis*) of our inner poisons during an inflammatory illness. Today we regard our inner work as a battle against a hostile virus or bacterium. The all-too-often overlooked point, however, is that it is we ourselves who inwardly, unconsciously determine whether or not to engage in the battle. The great medical pioneer Hans Selye, M.D., who introduced and elucidated the role of stress in health and illness, explained, "Disease is not mere surrender . . . but also fight for health; *unless there is fight there is no disease*" (emphasis mine).[1]

The symptoms of an acute inflammatory/infectious illness begin not when we are infected by a virus or bacterium, but when we respond. The magnitude of our response is influenced not only by the magnitude of the infection, but also by the inherent strength of what is responding in us. For the ancient physicians the responder in us was an aspect of our human spirit and our inner vitality, our inner healing force. Today the physical basis of our inner responder is what we call our immune system. The phenomenon of immunity hasn't changed, but our thinking about it has.

The severity of the early symptoms of a particular illness is directly proportional to the vigor of our immune response, and indirectly proportional to the burden and noxiousness of the infection to which we are responding. The surprising fact is that most of the symptoms of an infectious disease are caused not by the germs themselves but by our own activity of the immune system in fighting the germs. The germ "invasion" of our body is often silent, and can take place gradually over a long period of time without disturbing us. It is only when our immune system decides to do battle with the encroaching germs that we start to feel sick.

The metaphor of battle is a convenient but not fully accurate description of the relationship between our immune system and the proliferating viruses or bacteria during an acute inflammatory/infectious illness. Pasteur's germ theory assumes that

17

germs have a predatory nature: that they prey on our flesh for their own survival, while contributing nothing in return. The germ theory further assumes that the harmful or lethal effects of inflammatory/infectious diseases are a direct result of this "predation."

In early microscopic studies of host tissues in acute inflammatory/infectious diseases, Pasteur, Koch, and their colleagues repeatedly observed that germs were proliferating while many host cells were dying. They made the critical assumption that germs attack and destroy otherwise healthy cells, thus causing direct harm to the human body.

The observable facts would have equally justified the assumption that the host cells were dying for inapparent biochemical reasons, and that the proliferating germs were attracted to the site of increased cell death and decay just as flies, crows, and vultures are attracted to dead and dying animals. These early researchers had a choice between regarding germs as predators and regarding them as scavengers. The scientific world was captivated at the time by Darwinian images of "Nature red in tooth and claw" and the relentless struggle for survival. The perhaps inevitable choice of the "predator" model has made all the difference in our current thinking about illness and health. That early decision by Pasteur and his followers led to medicine's nearly exclusive focus on combating germs, while neglecting all the subtle but far-reaching ways of strengthening the host against lasting harm from inflammatory/infectious illness.

Like flies, crows, and vultures, which were regarded by the Native Americans as playing a necessary and helpful role in the great chain of Being, germs scavenge death and decay within our bodies. The true causes of inflammatory/infectious illnesses will ultimately be found to reside not in the germs but in the various human frailties that allow the forces of death and decay to predominate in us. The scavenging germs are the markers of our waxing and waning states of physiologic imbalance when cell death and decay temporarily exceed their normal limits.

The metaphor of battle between immune system and germs is justified provided we remember that our real enemies are the forces of death and decay. The germs themselves become sacrificial victims marked for destruction by our immune system because their role is to absorb the products of death and decay. Germs become poisonous to us by embodying the poisons we create. In "battling" germs, the real battle is to overcome ourselves and to refine our nature. This concept is implicit in the following discussion of how our immune system does battle with germs.

Using battle as our metaphor, we can imagine three possible scenarios. In the first, the attacking army is not strong, but the defenders are, and the attackers are routed from the field in a bloody but one-sided and brief battle in which the defenders suffer no casualties. This describes a typical case of a benign but acute inflammatory-infectious illness, like roseola, which usually expresses itself in a very high fever of 105 or 106 degrees and an extensive rash despite being no threat whatsoever to the host.

In the second scenario, the opposing armies are evenly matched, and there is a fierce battle with many casualties on both sides. This could describe an acute, life-threatening inflammatory illness, like septicemia or an overwhelming pneumonia, in which recovery or death is equally likely.

In the third scenario, the war reporter arrives late at the battlefield and finds no carnage, and little or no evidence of battle. The defending army is quiet and no attackers can be seen. The reporter at first concludes that it was a quick and easy victory for the defenders and that the attackers have fled. On closer investigation, however, one finds that no battle took place, because the defenders were unable or unwilling to fight. What our reporter at first thought was the defending army in reality consists of non-combatant defenders who have been quietly and massively infiltrated by the attackers. The attackers blend in, occupying the defenders' homeland, and any defenders who would fight them have gone underground, where they intermittently harass and provoke the occupying enemy.

The point of this elaborate metaphor is to demonstrate by analogy that the absence of fevers and other symptoms and signs of inflammatory illness (the battle) does not always mean that our immune system (the defending army) has been victorious! Today it is more often the case that when we don't fight our battles vigorously and often enough—when our fevers and discharging inflammations are very seldom and mild—then we are liable to be infiltrated by the enemy in disguise and to suffer from chronic allergic or autoimmune disorders. This concept today is called the hygiene hypothesis. In the 1920s Rudolf Steiner expounded essentially the same concept as an interplay between the opposing forces of inflammation and sclerosis, in which the healthy state is a dynamic balance between the two.

Returning to our third scenario, there are of course times when the absence of a battle, i.e., of obvious disease symptoms, indeed means that the defending army has easily routed the enemy and is truly immune from further attack. Thus we see that two entirely opposite outcomes, 1) immunity from attack, and 2) quiet infiltration by the attackers into the defender's homeland (the host body), can have *exactly the same appearance superficially*. This analogy also applies to another pair of similar-appearing but inwardly opposite states, i.e., the true immunity conferred by overcoming illness, and the apparent immunity conferred by vaccination. In both cases the host appears to be healthy due to the absence of illness, but true health is much more than the absence of overt illness. We will illustrate this point further in our discussion of smallpox below.

To complete our phenomenological description of immunity, we must note that in addition to the functions of clearing illnesses from the body and of recognizing the illnesses it has previously encountered, the immune system has another cognitive or knowing capacity. This is the discrimination of self from nonself and the ability to "tolerate," i.e., to not react to as foreign, any elements of self. This remarkable knowing of the immune system also extends to its ability to tolerate, in pregnancy, a massive foreign presence in the body, the fetus, without reacting to it at all.

Thus we see the incredible skill and apparent purposefulness of *doing* and the discriminating capacity of *knowing* possessed by the immune system. Although modern science rarely uses the words "knowing" and "doing" in its descriptions of the immune system, nevertheless distinct knowing and doing functions are clearly and unavoidably implied in all scientific writing on immunology. Science prefers to focus on the molecular level, hoping to find in molecular events the elusive key to understanding, if not why, at least *how* the immune system does what it does.

Today the immune system is most often described in articles and textbooks as comprising those bodily organs, cells, and functions which discriminate between self and non-self. The molecules of self or non-self that the immune system can recognize are called antigens. One branch of the immune system, called the humoral immune system, consists primarily of antibodies, which are protein molecules made by the body to specifically interact with foreign antigens. Antibodies attach themselves to any foreign antigens, like bacteria or parasites, that may exist in blood or body fluids outside of the body's cells, usually coating these antigens as one step in the complex process of the destruction, digestion, and elimination of foreign matter by our immune system.

We come now to a beginner's question, one seldom or never asked in the science of immunology: Why does our immune system work in such an inconsistent way, providing permanent immunity from recurrence after certain illnesses but not after others? A "why" question such as this is usually considered irrelevant in modern science, while the equivalent "how" question is actively pursued. In the case of immunity to illness, it is the "how" questions that have led science to the idea and the practice of vaccination.

For science, the pertinent question is: How can we imitate nature and bring about lifelong immunity to an infectious-inflammatory illness without having to experience the illness first? The first task would be to learn exactly how nature itself manages to maintain permanent immunity in us after a first experience of illness.

Part Two: How Does Vaccination Work?

Sometimes a practical scientific breakthrough happens out of an intuition, a hunch, long before the discoverer or anyone else is able to explain just how and why the discovery works. This is true of the work of Jenner and Pasteur, the great initiators of the practice of vaccination. Astoundingly, in our modern era, when vaccinations are so widely acclaimed and practiced, science still cannot explain how they work.

In the *New Scientist* (May 27, 2000), an article on AIDS vaccine research quotes two scientists: "I'm amazed by the amount of basic science we don't know," and "The assumption that successful vaccines work by simply producing antibodies is almost certainly wrong." The article then describes how one vaccine researcher found that in a certain viral disease of horses, while vaccination was successful in inducing antibodies against the virus, the vaccinated horses died faster than the unvaccinated ones. Referring to our present ignorance as to why these vaccinated horses succumbed, the scientist stated, "It's an issue people haven't wanted to think about, but we might have to."

Vaccine science and practice have always been based on certain assumptions that we are only now beginning to examine. One of these is that antibodies in the blood (humoral immunity) confer protection against an illness, and that the level of antibodies correlates with the degree of protection. This relationship between measurable antibodies in the blood and apparent protection from illness has been observed for decades in many types of infectious diseases. It is not known, however, whether the antibodies persisting in the blood for months or years after an infectious disease are themselves responsible for protecting us from recurrences of that disease, or whether they are merely markers of a protection that is accomplished by another part of the immune system. It is also not known whether the apparent protection associated with vaccination-induced antibodies is a benefit pure and simple or whether a hidden cost to the immune system is involved. The idea of a hidden cost is considered unthinkable by vaccine researchers for obvious practical reasons, yet it continues to be a nagging doubt among an ever-widening circle of parents, consumer advocates, chiropractors, holistic physicians, and other discerning people.

The vaccine research quoted above suggests that it's not the antibodies but the cellular immune system that protects us. Also called the cell-mediated immune system, it comprises the white blood cells and all the lymph nodes and lymphatic tissue throughout the body, and is concentrated in the thymus, tonsils, adenoids, spleen, and bone marrow. It is generally agreed that the primary function of the cellular immune system is to destroy foreign intracellular antigens, such as viruses and some bacteria, as well as the cells that harbor them. This is accomplished by the various white blood cells that are able to move inside, outside, and through the walls of our blood vessels and to access every part of the body.

In the past I thought to assign the immune system's doing function to the cell-mediated branch and its knowing function to the humoral antibody-mediated branch. This neat division of function is not borne out by the facts. Research shows us that each branch participates in functions of both knowing and doing, although most of the immune system's power to destroy, digest, and drive out intruders comes from its cell-mediated branch. Thus, while immune system functions of knowing and doing may be conceptually distinct, in the physical reality they are overlapping in an exceedingly complex orchestration of organs, cells, molecules, hormones, and chemical messengers.[2]

At the present time, it is thought that the encounter between self and non-self, that is, between the immune system and a foreign "invader" such as a virus or bacterium, begins in the domain of the cellular immune system. If the foreign guests are not great in number or in noxiousness, the cellular immune system is able to dispatch them, digest them, and clear them from the body without ever calling into action its coworker, the humoral or antibody-mediated immune system. We are continually infected with many small numbers of different germs, some of them nasty, and the cells of our immune system continually shepherd them and keep them in check, without our awareness and without the assistance of antibodies.

Like dust and other unseen debris, these microorganisms enter our bodies as we breathe, eat, and drink. Only when the number or growth rate of germs exceeds a certain threshold are they recognized by the humoral immune system, resulting in the formation of antibodies specific to the particular provocative bug. At this stage we may have only mild, fleeting symptoms, or none at all. This explains how we may be found to have antibodies against illnesses we don't remember ever having had! The phenomenon is called "subclinical infection," i.e., infection without symptoms, and it happens commonly.

Science has discerned three levels of infection. The lowest level is the aforementioned steady-state equilibrium of everyday life, in which we peacefully co-exist with our inner menagerie of germs without needing to form detectable antibodies against them. At this lowest level our cellular immune system is quietly busy keeping our bugs in line and, when necessary, culling the herd. Thus, although small numbers of disease agents are within us, our cellular immune system sees to it that we remain well and free of disease symptoms, and that our germs are under control.

At the second level of infection, we temporarily relax our vigilance and allow a certain group of germs to begin rapidly multiplying to the point where the humoral immune system is alerted and begins to produce antibodies against the offending bugs. This sets off a cascade of immune system functions, which succeed in quelling our rebelling germs so quickly that the person hosting all these inner happenings is unaware of having just gone through a subclinical illness. The identity of the wayward germ can afterwards be diagnosed by the presence in the blood serum of the specific antibodies produced against it by the humoral immune system.

At the third level of infection, things get seriously out of control, and all our inner alarm bells go off as a tribe of germs proliferates wildly and provokes the full defensive reaction of our immune system. This is called the "acute inflammatory response" and usually includes fever; release of stress hormones by the adrenal glands; increased flow of blood, lymph, and mucus; and a streaming of white blood cells to the inflamed area. The human host of these wisdom-filled events now feels sick and may experience pain, nausea, vomiting, diarrhea, weakness, chills, and fever. We have now emerged from the realm of the subclinical to a full-blown clinical illness, with all of its intense and often frightening symptoms.

It is critical to a healthy understanding of this process to realize that we never merely suffer through an illness in a passive, one-dimensional way. In an acute illness, parts of us that in health are most active, like our mind and our muscles, are subdued, while other parts, like our blood, glands, and immune system, are much more active than normal. Thus every illness rouses us to become more inwardly active than usual, and this inner activity of ours is the cooking through, the sweating out, and the throwing off of the illness. This is hard work, and every illness calls upon and exercises capacities in us that otherwise would have remained dormant. Adults often notice these new capacities as a change in attitude or outlook after an illness. Children often manifest positive changes in their behavior or development after overcoming an acute inflammation or fever.

Having successfully passed the challenge of a particular illness, we may not need to experience it again. Something about the illness and our response to it has made us immune to its recurrence. If we knew what that something was, perhaps we could learn how to use it to create health and prevent illness. Of course, this is the basic concept of vaccination, but the all-important question is, does vaccination accomplish what we think it does?

We've already suggested that it's primarily the cellular immune system, and not antibodies, that protect us against illness. Surely antibodies can have little or no role in either preventing or overcoming first bouts of infectious-inflammatory illness, because they are formed only after the illness has peaked. It must be the cellular immune system that confers the resistance to, as well as the capacity to overcome, both first episodes and subsequent episodes of infectious disease. To understand how this might happen, it is helpful to examine more closely the very illness and vaccination that started the whole debate: smallpox.

Part Three: Smallpox and Its Vaccination

That vaccines can confer a degree of protection from certain infectious-inflammatory illnesses is clear. What is not clear is exactly what vaccinations do to the immune system to bring about their protective effect. Researchers generally agree that vaccines do not prevent the particular virus or bacterium from entering the body or from beginning to multiply within it. It is thought instead that the vaccines stimulate or "prime" the immune system to quickly eradicate the offending germ soon after it begins to infect the host.

Let us consider how this process might work in the case of smallpox. Our knowledge about smallpox and its vaccination is based on over two hundred years of study of this dramatic and much-feared illness by physicians in many countries.

The natural course of the illness begins when one "catches" smallpox from someone with a smallpox rash or from the mucus or pus on an afflicted patient's bedclothes or dressings. For the next twelve days, there are no signs or symptoms at all, and the new patient is not contagious, even though the smallpox virus is multiplying within the body. On or about the twelfth day, large numbers of smallpox virus enter the blood (viremia) and the "toxemic" phase of the illness begins, meaning a poisoning or contamination of the blood. This blood poisoning is the beginning of the overt illness, with symptoms of fever, prostration, severe headache, backache, limb pains, and sometimes vomiting.

After three or four days of these symptoms, the typical smallpox rash begins to erupt, and in the next one to two days the fever falls to almost normal and the patient feels much better.

The skin eruption begins as red spots that over the next few days evolve into raised pimples, then change to blisters and fill with pus. On the eleventh to the thirteenth day of the illness, the pustules begin to dry up and form crusts or scabs, which fall off by the end of the third week of the illness. The fever usually returns, less severely, after the pustules appear, and departs as the crusts and scabs form. While a person may die in the first week of the illness if the toxemia is very severe, most smallpox deaths have occurred toward the end of the second week, after the pustules appear.

The majority of smallpox patients survive, and the falling away of the dried-up scabs from the skin signifies the final stage of healing, approximately thirty-three days after catching the infection. The dramatic course of smallpox illustrates very well some of the concepts discussed above. The twelve-day incubation period during which the smallpox virus actively multiplies in the body without provoking the slightest symptom confirms the point that it is our response to infection, not the infection itself, that causes the typical disease symptoms of fever, aches and pains, and extreme weakness.

The fact that the fever drops and the patient feels much better after the rash breaks out illustrates Hering's law. The poisons circulating in the blood during the toxemic phase cause the most severe symptoms of smallpox. These symptoms improve considerably once the blood clears out its poisons by discharging them through the skin, producing the typical pus-filled blisters of smallpox. The chief danger of smallpox consists in the degree of blood poisoning and in the huge and exhausting effort required for the immune system to push the poisons out of the blood and through the skin. When the poisons are overwhelming and the patient lacks the strength to discharge them, then the patient may die in the effort, either before the eruption ever appears or else, utterly spent, afterwards.

The patients who survive smallpox will have lifelong neutralizing antibodies to smallpox virus in their blood and permanent immunity to a second episode of the illness. What does this mean?

Using the battle metaphor, we could say that the victorious defending army has acquired much valuable skill, know-how, and confidence through its combat experience, in addition to certain medals awarded to acknowledge its participation in combat. The first three attributes are comparable to the inner strengthening of the cellular immune system that is attained through overcoming an illness like smallpox. The medals, as visible tokens of achievement, are roughly comparable to the antibodies visible on simple blood tests indicating that the host has already won that battle and is likely to be immune to future attacks of the same illness.

If a foolish general were under the illusion that merely wearing a combat medal actually conferred the know-how, skill, and confidence gained in battle, then he might propose pinning medals on soldiers with no combat experience to make them immune to dangerous future battles. That would bestow the same outward appearance on seasoned and unseasoned soldiers alike, belying their experience.

In the same way, science bestows antibodies through vaccination and mistakenly assumes that it is bestowing the immune strength that can only be developed through the experience of illness. In equating the significance of vaccine-induced antibodies with that of illness-induced antibodies, science confuses the outer sign of the battle experience with the experience itself.

Antibodies arising through illness are markers of immunity and (unlike the medals in our battle metaphor) also contribute to immunity, but antibodies alone are not sufficient to confer lasting immunity to a particular illness. There are several diseases that may recur repeatedly, such as herpes outbreaks, despite high antibody levels. The evidence suggests that it is our cellular immune system that confers lasting immunity, with antibodies playing a secondary role in the process.

Immunity is really the result of our experience, of having gone through, along with our cellular immune system, an *active process* (the combat in the metaphor) of learning and strengthening. The immune system is not a self-contained mechanism. It is an aspect of who we are as human beings, and as we learn from experience, our immune system learns, too. Antibodies signify that we've had experience, often repeatedly, but not necessarily that we've gained anything from the experience. When on some level we respond with greater initiative to our experience of illness, actively processing, digesting, and ultimately learning from such experience, then we are usually immune from having to repeat it. In such cases, our cellular immune system has strengthened itself through its active encounter with, and vanquishing of, the illness. In this view, immunity is the result of having successfully met the challenge of a particular illness and gained mastery over it. It is like learning a skill, such as riding a bicycle, that is retained for life. On the physiologic level, the skill and mastery we gain in overcoming illness accrue to our cellular immune system.

This active process of acquiring mastery cannot be replaced by a vaccination unless the host's immune response to the vaccination is essentially identical to its response to the illness itself, even though reduced in intensity. This would mean that in order to produce genuine cellular immunity, a vaccination would have to reproduce the experience of the illness, causing some of the same signs and symptoms (though milder) that are caused by the illness. To see if this is true, let us look at smallpox vaccination.

The vaccination consists of introducing live cowpox (vaccinia) virus into the skin by multiple superficial punctures in a small area about one-eighth of an inch in diameter on the upper arm. The vaccination site is then inspected after three and nine days to determine whether the vaccination "takes" or not. A primary reaction or "take" evolves as follows: for three days after the vaccination, there is no reaction. On the fourth day, a small red pimple appears, which gradually grows into a blister, then a pustule surrounded by a zone of redness. There is often a mild fever and tender, swollen glands in the armpit. This reaction peaks on the eighth to the tenth day, after which the pustule gradually dries up and forms a scab that leaves a scar when it falls off.

Clearly, the primary "take" reproduces the experience of smallpox itself described earlier, but in a very limited way, so as to generate only one pock rather than many dozens of them. The cellular immunity produced by smallpox vaccination is also limited, lasting from six months to three years. This immunity probably coincides with the length of time that the exercised "muscle" of the cellular immune system remains strengthened from its labor of discharging the single cow pock resulting from the vaccination. The antibodies appearing in the blood after primary smallpox vaccination may remain for over ten years, but these antibodies cannot be taken as a trustworthy sign of immunity. The official description of the currently available smallpox vaccine in the U.S., which was manufactured by Wyeth Laboratories, states that "the level of antibody that protects against smallpox infection is unknown."[3] If we can state blandly that the protective level of antibody is still unknown after having assumed for several decades that protection is directly correlated with antibody level, then surely it is time to rethink that assumption.

In the smallpox era, antibody levels were seldom used in practice as a measure of immunity. Anyone not vaccinated in the previous three years was considered to be susceptible to smallpox, regardless of the person's antibody level.

The all-important question is how to interpret the meaning of reactions to smallpox vaccination that are milder and briefer than the primary "take"—which does result in a genuine though short-lived immunity of the cell-mediated system.

Since the early 1970s only two types of reactions to smallpox vaccination have been officially recognized, as recommended by the World Health Organization (WHO). For purposes of greater clarity, in this discussion I will be referring to the older classification, which recognized three types of normal reactions to smallpox vaccination.

The second type of normal skin reaction was called the accelerated or vaccinoid reaction, usually occurring in people who had some immunity to smallpox at the time of vaccination, either from a previous experience of the disease or from a previous smallpox vaccination. In the accelerated reaction, the skin blister is smaller and reaches its maximum size and intensity between the third and the seventh day after the vaccination. This reaction works in exactly the same way as the primary reaction but to a lesser degree, boosting the cell-mediated immunity that is already present, but waning, from the previous vaccination.

It is the third type of reaction to smallpox vaccination that in my opinion has created all the problems and has been at the root of a two-hundred-year-old controversy over the usefulness of smallpox vaccination. This stems from the fact that this reaction for years was interpreted as indicating immunity to smallpox, when often it meant exactly the opposite. In many cases, the bearers of this reaction may have had a suppressed cellular immunity, making them on repeated revaccination more susceptible to smallpox than an unvaccinated person!

This third type of reaction was originally called an immune reaction and was later renamed an early or immediate reaction. A small pimple forms at the vaccination site that may evolve into a tiny blister, peaking on the second or third day and diminishing thereafter. An earlier textbook of viral diseases from the smallpox era states: "The early or immediate reaction is an indication of sensitivity to the virus . . . by persons *who are either susceptible or immune to smallpox*. . . . [It] cannot be regarded as a successful result and cannot be guaranteed to induce or increase the person's resistance to smallpox" (emphasis mine).[4] This is a typical scientific understatement that glosses over years of devastating results of smallpox vaccination in which thousands of vaccinated people who were thought to be immune based on their so-called "immune reaction" to vaccination later caught smallpox and died.

Ian Sinclair, writing on the history of smallpox, states:

> After an intensive four-year effort to vaccinate the entire population between the ages of 2 and 50, the Chief Medical Officer of England announced in May 1871 that 97.5% had been vaccinated. In the following year, 1872, England experienced its worst ever smallpox epidemic which claimed 44,840 lives. . . . In the Philippines, prior to U.S. takeover in 1905, case mortality [death rate] from smallpox was about 10%. . . . In 1918–1919, with over 95% of the population vaccinated, the worst epidemic in the Philippines' history occurred resulting in a case mortality of 65%. . . . The 1920 Report of the Philippines Health Service [stated] . . . "hundreds of

thousands of people were yearly vaccinated with the most unfortunate result that the 1918 epidemic looks prima facie as a flagrant failure of the classic immunization toward future epidemics."[5]

How can this be? How can these historical facts be reconciled with my earlier statement that a primary "take" in response to a first smallpox vaccination results in genuine cellular immunity for up to three years? The usual explanation offered is that the vaccine used was inactive due to loss of potency in storage, but this clearly cannot be the whole answer to the many documented instances of failure of smallpox vaccination to protect from smallpox.

The answer is an open secret that has been very well known for years but never fully understood: that many first recipients of smallpox vaccine fail to produce a "take" (primary reaction) and continue to fail to do so even when revaccinated many times. The textbook states,

Easton (1945) records of one man who died of confluent smallpox that vaccination had been attempted at birth, again in 1941 and ten times in 1943 without a take, thus emphasizing the danger of accepting even repeated unsuccessful vaccination as evidence of insusceptibility to smallpox.[6]

This is an excellent example of a vitally important observation leading to an irrelevant, though not incorrect, conclusion. This example begs the question: How many repeated failures to react does it take to justify the concern that continuing to revaccinate may be doing more harm than good?

★ ★ ★

The relevant conclusion, in my opinion, is that due to differences in immune response capability among individual human
beings at the time of first vaccination, in some individuals the
cellular immune system lacks the muscle to push out the single
pock eruption that is the primary take. The scratching of the
virus into the skin of the arm is a strong challenge to the
immune system. A successful take depends on the ability of the
cellular immune system to respond to that challenge in an equally vigorous way, to push the intruding virus right back out of the
body. It is a simple matter of action and reaction, of challenge
and response. If Charles Atlas challenges a ninety-seven-pound
weakling to arm wrestling and his opponent's arm immediately
collapses, we would not think that the challenge ought to be
repeated indefinitely if the weak condition of the responder had
no means of improving! Yet in thousands of individuals in the last
two hundred years who may have been weakened by stress, poor
nutrition, and poverty, whose cellular immune systems were not
vigorous enough to respond to smallpox vaccination with a
"take," the effect of repeated revaccination, which was commonly practiced, was to weaken these individuals' immune systems
still further, making them no doubt more vulnerable to smallpox
than they had been before vaccination! This would explain the
disastrous results of the above-mentioned smallpox vaccination
campaigns in England and the Philippines, and in many other
countries as well.

The ambivalent nature of the so-called early or immediate
reaction to smallpox vaccination is analogous to the third battle
scenario mentioned earlier in this article. When few or no signs
of battle (reaction) are visible, it may mean that the defenders
were easily victorious (the host is immune), or it may mean that

the defenders lacked the strength to fight and their homeland was subsequently quietly infiltrated by the attackers. When a smallpox vaccine recipient lacks the immune muscle to respond to the viral intrusion of his or her body with a vigorous pock-forming discharge, then we might expect that most of the intruding virus has remained in the body. With each revaccination the burden of vaccinia virus in the body increases, and the suppressive effect of this viral burden on the cellular immune system also increases, eventually resulting in a dangerous state of immunosuppression. This may also explain the occasionally catastrophic effects that were observed resulting from a brief medical fad in the 1970s: treating recurrent herpes infections with repeated smallpox vaccinations.

Smallpox and its vaccination are fruitful subjects to study in order to understand how the immune system works, because we can observe what happens on the skin as vital clues to what might be happening inside the body. The main lesson from this study is that a lack of a vaccine reaction, and by extension *a lack of illness symptoms, can by no means be taken as a sign of immunity or of health.*

The other critical fact confirmed by our historical experience with smallpox vaccination is that individual differences in response to vaccination are extremely important. One size most definitely does not fit all. It is clear that although the smallpox vaccine was effective in conferring a temporary immunity in some individuals, an unknown number of other individuals were probably harmed by the vaccine. The same vaccination procedure that temporarily strengthened the cellular immune system in some people no doubt weakened it in others, especially upon repeated revaccination. Adverse effects of the vaccine were fairly obvious, often appearing on the skin, but with other vaccines in use today the adverse effects may not be so obvious.

★ ★ ★

The possibility that the up to thirty-seven doses of eleven
different vaccines that children today receive by the time they
start school may be impacting the cellular immune systems of
many individual children in a negative way, suggests itself to the
open mind. Science has most of the knowledge and the tools it
needs to investigate and to find answers to these unanswered
questions. All it needs now is the will. May it come soon, for our
children's sake.

1. Selye, Hans. *The Stress of Life.* New York: McGraw-Hill, 1978,
    p. 12.
2. There are also other aspects of the immune system that are
    beyond the scope of this article. Reading a modern textbook
    of immunology can be frustrating, as one finds a bewildering
    array of cellular, molecular, and antibody-mediated processes
    that science has discovered without knowing how they all fit
    together and manage to cooperate in health and in illness in
    the human being. It's something like trying to understand
    how an automobile performs by studying its disassembled
    parts in an auto parts shop.
3. Centers for Disease Control, *Morbidity and Mortality Weekly
    Report,* June 22, 2001, Vol. 50, No. RR-10.
4. Rivers, T. M., and F. L. Horsfall, Jr. *Viral and Rickettsial Infections
    of Man.* Philadelphia: Lippincott, 1959, p. 686.
5. In *Vaccination: The "Hidden" Facts* by Ian Sinclair, 5 Ivy St,
    Ryde NSW 2112, Australia.
6. Rivers and Horsfall, p. 687.

✍ Taking Your Child to an Anthroposophic Doctor

Mary Kelly Sutton, M.D.

To discuss immunization fruitfully, one must find balance and be willing to educate oneself about each disease and each immunization. There is a touch of hysteria in the common literature both for and against standard immunization recommendations. Often, recommendations emphasize the problems with the disease without thoroughly listing the possible adverse reactions to the vaccine.

The single most valuable balanced source of information I have found is the National Vaccine Information Center (see Resource pages). Barbara Loe Fisher, the president of NVIC, has a son who was brain-damaged by the diphtheria, pertussis, and tetanus (DPT) vaccine, and a relative who suffered residual damage from pertussis (whooping cough). She knows the risks of vaccinating and not vaccinating, and speaks with awareness and balance. Through her work the National Vaccine Adverse Event Reporting System was established. Though it is estimated that only one to ten percent of adverse reactions to vaccines are reported, there are still over a thousand reports per month.

The creation of public health immunization programs in each state is based on preventing illnesses, some of which are serious illnesses and some of which are acute illnesses common to childhood. In seeking the public good, medical organizations, allied with government, have created a schedule of immunization that allows for the greatest possible number of children to be immunized. This is public-health thinking—the medicine of numbers and populations—and sometimes is in contrast to what is optimum care for an individual. By definition, current programs aimed at mass immunization do not distinguish among the differing degrees of risk posed by each disease. For example, all newborns get hepatitis B vaccine in the standard protocol, even if there is no family member or contact with the disease. And it is uncommon to find physicians who screen patients in order to avoid reactions to immunization.

More and more, the call to awareness is coming to the medical profession from the parents themselves. Parents are seeking to individualize their children's care in a way that respects who the child is as an individual. Did the infant have an easy delivery, or was jaundice, poor nursing, or long labor a problem? Parents and some doctors are wont to administer immunizations in identical fashion to children who have very different genetic backgrounds and medical history. There are those who object to giving immediate immunization to any newborn, even one in vigorous health, simply because the child is not yet fully known, and is undergoing an enormous transition from watery darkness into air and light, from total non-breathing dependence on the mother's placenta, to breathing, movement, suckling, and the beginning world of the senses. "Is this a time for an immunization?" some rightfully ask. The magnitude of the moment is jarred by an invasive event. At times the health of the infant requires an early vaccine (such as if a family member has an active disease), but this should not be a routine for each baby entering the world.

For the family of each infant, I provide a folder with the standard information on vaccines, a statement by a medical doctor on involving parents in decision-making about vaccines, and the contact numbers for the NVIC. When a parent has read about each vaccine and disease, I ask about the baby's circumstances and family history. Is there a history of reactions to vaccines in the baby or in family members? Is there neurologic or autoimmune disease, including autism or Attention Deficit Hyperactivity Disorder (ADHD), in the family? What is the risk to the baby posed by the disease we are discussing vaccinating against? The answer could be influenced by seasonal diseases, the presence of siblings who attend school, the nature and location of the parents' work. What is the baby's current state of health? Is travel planned? What is the parents' degree of emotional comfort in dealing with either a disease or a vaccination?

An important question to ask is, "How would you feel if your child caught ___?" If the answer is one of panic and heavy guilt, then the immunization is better than the disease, because of the emotional weight the parent would carry. If the answer is, "It would be tough, but we'd get through," then skipping the immunization may be an option.

A couple of important changes in immunization practice have occurred. Oral polio vaccine is no longer recommended. Though this vaccine is a mimic of the natural disease, ingesting it orally has the downside of creating a pool of virus-shedding children for about six weeks after each dose. This is not a problem generally in older children who control their stool, but has been a problem among infants and toddlers who might have accidents. Fecal-oral contamination has inadvertently allowed the vaccine virus to cause some cases of polio regularly each year. Now, the injectable polio vaccine is used. This virus is dead, and no risk of spread of polio is known to occur.

With all injectables we bypass the natural barrier of the skin and the purity of the product becomes paramount. Recently, concern about thimerosal as a preservative in vaccines has stimulated the vaccine industry to offer a diphtheria, tetanus, and pertussis vaccine (DTaP) without mercury (thimerosal) preservative. Research seeks to determine if tiny mercury doses early in life are related to autism or ADHD.

Some parents choose to separate vaccines into one-at-a-time administration. I knew a Pakistani physician in the Emirates who said she would never consider administering an measles, mumps, and rubella (MMR) vaccine to her patients; she gave measles separate from mumps, separate from rubella. Perhaps a modest work load for the immune system is less likely to induce adverse effects than many antigens at one sitting.

Unfortunately, more money is spent on research and development than on the basic research needed to understand why adverse reactions happen and what role nutrition or timing might play. The research leading to the development of new vaccines results in more economic gain, of course, while the basic science research gives purely human benefit.

Parents should inform themselves fully so they can feel satisfied that they have delved into both sides. Each disease and each immunization must be considered, and reconsidered. While a family may decide not to immunize with MMR at fifteen months and five years, the family may choose to immunize against one or all three diseases when the child reaches adolescence. Mumps in a pubertal male can settle into a testicle, and loss of fertility in that testicle can occur. Rubella endured in the first trimester of pregnancy can cause hearing loss in the developing fetus.

In most states, people become responsible for their own fate at the age of eighteen, at which time they should be told what immunizations they have had. At this point, judgment is again called into play to determine the need for further immunizations, based on the health of the individual and the risk expected. Joining the Peace Corps would, for example, likely require more immunizations.

This is the kind of individualized medicine parents are seeking. What is required is a thorough look at the individual, and some consideration of the context in which the immunization is used.

Part II

How to Treat Childhood Illnesses

❧ Common Childhood Illnesses

Michaela Gloecker, M.D., and Wolfgang Goebel, M.D.

In countries all over the world it is now normal practice to immunize the very young against tuberculosis, tetanus, diptheria, polio, measles, mumps, whooping cough, and other illnesses. As a result there is a tendency for people to believe that children's diseases are not to be endured at all. Yet feverish illnesses present the child's organism with a chance to develop and strengthen itself, overcoming hereditary influences unsuited to the child's own personality and building up a well-functioning immune system. Although there is occasional risk that an illness might leave permanent damage, damage may equally well be caused by the wrong treatment, for example, the indiscriminate use of antipyretics (fever-reducing drugs).

The following is a brief account of the most common children's illnesses, describing their normal course. It is assumed that you already have a physician who is willing to assist you through the childhood illnesses you may encounter. He or she should be at your side from the beginning, supervising the course of the illness. Quarantine rules must be followed.

Childhood illnesses often announce themselves in advance as a certain restlessness or malaise. When your child begins to be acutely unwell, contact your doctor immediately. If an infectious illness is suspected, do not take the child to the waiting room or hospital, but ask for instructions. Most feverish childhood illnesses have the same basic requirements: warm bed rest, liquids, and restricted diet.

In our experience, a child kept in bed through an illness, nursed with love and care and given a chance to convalesce afterwards, is better able to cope with common childhood ailments. Generally speaking, the homeopathic or anthroposophical physician will prescribe only those medicines which strengthen the organism, rather than those which merely suppress symptoms, unless a complication during the course of the illness necessitates more stringent measures.

After the illness and a good convalescence, parents can often observe a positive change: a spurt in growth, a more individual facial expression, new abilities, new interests, and a greater stability in general health. One nine-year old girl exclaimed in surprise after one of these illnesses: "The whole world looks freshly washed!" She felt herself newborn and at the beginning of a new phase of development.

MEASLES

Measles is a common infectious disease found all over the world, mainly in preschool children. Nearly all children are susceptible, although in the Westernized world cases are rare due to immunization programs. If the disease is contracted as an adult, it is usually more severe than in childhood.

Symptoms
The illness starts with a harmless cold, slightly reddened eyes, and a loose cough. A slight fever may develop, followed by a temporary improvement for a day or two. The first signs of measles are

in the child's mouth: little white spots and stripes on the inside of the cheeks. On the fourth day, the child will begin to feel cold and develop a high fever. At the same time, the characteristic rash appears, with merging spots beginning behind the ears and head, spreading quickly over the arms and legs. After three more days the child will generally be feeling much better but may continue to have a cough for a week or more. The parents should stay in touch with the physician at all times, especially if the fever has not subsided after three days or if there have been further developments, such as earache or vomiting.

Treatment

This illness runs a fairly typical course. Children with measles just want to rest and should be kept in bed and provided with plenty of liquids. They are likely to hide away under the blankets, avoiding the light. Listless and disinclined to talk, they are prone to a loose cough with mucus. Their faces are red-spotted and bloated, with the eyes swollen to slits, making seeing difficult. Keep the sickroom quiet, with little or low light.

Complications

The most common complications of measles are pneumonia, inflammation of the middle ear (purulent otitis media), and sinusitis. Febrile convulsions at the beginning of the illness normally cause no lasting harm. The greatest danger following a bout of measles is the possibility of encephalitis, which is indicated by renewed fever after the rash has faded, with delirium and possibly convulsions. A child with encephalitis must be hospitalized as soon as possible. At the beginning of the 1960s, the frequency of measles encephalitis in West Germany was reckoned to be 1:14,500. The latest figures available are 1:1,000 to 1:2,000. We believe that this increased frequency may well result from the routine use of antipyretics. Considering the important part played by fever in combating the virus that causes the illness, this possibility cannot be overlooked. Children who have not had suppressive treatments for previous infectious illnesses are likely to recover from measles better than children who have.

GERMAN MEASLES (RUBELLA)

In children, German measles is generally a harmless illness. It is not related to ordinary measles and is not as infectious. The principal risk is to expectant mothers. If a woman without immunity is in contact with German measles during the first four months of pregnancy, her child may miscarry or be born with malformations.

Symptoms

Two to three weeks after infection, a rash appears, sometimes followed by a fever. Characteristically, the lymph nodes around the neck, throat, and back of the head become swollen. At first sight, the rash is similar to that of measles, but the spots are more evenly distributed over the body, though concentrating on the trunk, and tend not to merge. The fever can be high but is fairly uncomplicated.

Exposure

Without immunization, eighty to ninety percent of children who catch the disease before the age of twenty acquire immunity, or else they become immune through subclinical infection (meaning that the body has overcome the infection without becoming overtly ill). Whether or not a child has acquired immunity can be ascertained by a blood test. In many countries, immunization is recommended before puberty for all girls who have not had German measles.

Treatment
Keep the child in bed and provide plenty of liquids as long as the fever lasts.

SCARLET FEVER

After an incubation period of two to five days, the child breaks out in a fever rising sharply to 102 to 105 degrees and feels very unwell, perhaps vomiting and shivering. The diagnosis may be confirmed by taking a throat swab to test for streptococcus bacteria.

Symptoms
The tongue has a heavy white coating and the back of the throat and tonsils turn red. The child may complain of a sore throat. The nasal membranes may be affected, but there is not as much phlegm as with measles. In typical cases the cheeks are dark red, but with a characteristic pale triangle around the mouth. The rash normally appears on the trunk but may show only at the groin, lower belly, and thighs. From a distance the rash appears to be a uniformly reddened area gradually diminishing towards the edges. Close up, the fine single spots look like goose bumps. While in measles the face is swollen and damp, in scarlet fever it is more clear-cut and dry.

After two to three days the coating on the tongue peels off, leaving a "raspberry tongue" with fine papules. After another one to three days the fever dies down. The last sign of scarlet fever is peeling skin on the hands and feet after about two weeks. Keep your child in bed for at least three weeks and provide plenty of liquids. At the end of the quarantine period, the patient should be given a thorough bath.

Complications
Nowadays the course of the illness is nearly always harmless, even
without antibiotics. Occasionally it may leave pus-pimples with
scabs around the mouth, or an inflammation of the middle ear,
both of which should be treated by a doctor. The more serious
complications that were once so feared, such as rheumatic fever
or inflammation of the heart and kidneys, have become very rare
in recent years. Even so, scarlet fever in its classic form must be
regarded as a catabolic illness (one that breaks down substances
of the body), affecting and possibly damaging the vital organs.
Hence it is strongly recommended that the illness be followed by
at least three weeks of strict convalescence, during which time
the child must be spared any exertion. During this period the
doctor will continue various checks and tests. Unlike measles,
recurrences of scarlet fever can occur. In our experience this
happens much more frequently after cases in which antibiotics
were prescribed.

DIPHTHERIA
Diphtheria, a highly contagious disease, is now very rare in
Western countries; it had started to decline even before immunization was widespread. Yet at the beginning of last century, it
was still called "the children's angel of death."

Symptoms
Two to five days after catching the infection, the patient develops a sore throat and hoarseness, sometimes with fever. A dirty
white coating extends over and beyond the tonsils. The symptoms are quite distinct from other upper respiratory illnesses. The
patient is often pale, without high fever but with a quick, soft
pulse and a tendency to low blood pressure, swollen lymph
nodes, inflammation of the mucous membranes, and a character-

istic sweetish smell in the mouth. The symptoms reflect a toxic state that particularly affects the nervous and circulatory systems. At its worst it can lead to weakening of the heart muscles, collapse, and paralysis.

Treatment
Treatment of diphtheria nearly always has to be in the hospital with diphtheria serum and antibiotics.

CHICKEN POX
This airborne illness is extremely contagious and mostly affects children under the age of ten. The incubation period is thirteen to twenty-one days.

Symptoms
Over a few days, small spots appear irregularly over the body, like a map of the heavens. These quickly grow into watery blisters, about an eighth of an inch across, which become covered with crusts. The blisters appear under the hair of the head, on the hands, in the mouth, and on the genitals. Pains in the stomach indicate that the intestinal membranes have been affected. The blisters on the outer skin are not painful, but they are itchy and the patient is inclined to scratch. There may be fever, but it is usually of short duration. During the fever the child should be kept in bed, but if there is no fever, bed rest is not necessary.

Treatment
Treatment is usually limited to whatever can be done to reduce the itching. Telling your child to stop scratching will usually have the opposite effect! A soothing powder with an anti-itch ingredient or a lukewarm bath with chamomile infusion or pine bath lotion may help. If pus has formed in the blisters, some scars may

remain, but the smaller ones usually disappear over the course of time.

Exposure

Chicken pox is infectious from two days before the appearance and crusting over of the blisters to one week afterward. As the disease is much more contagious than measles, children may be kept home from school until the skin has completely cleared.

Chicken pox can be dangerous for newborn infants if they have not acquired immunity through their mothers. If you think your baby may have been exposed to chicken pox, consult your doctor without delay.

Chicken pox and shingles

A few people exposed to chicken pox may be inclined in later life to get shingles (*herpes zoster*), a related illness caused by the same virus. Children can be infected by an adult with shingles and develop chicken pox. In shingles, groups of blisters appear in lines or clusters on one side of the face, trunk, or limbs. The blisters are often accompanied by pain and a sustained high fever.

MUMPS (EPIDEMIC PAROTITIS)

Children usually catch mumps after the age of five. There is an incubation period of approximately two to three weeks before symptoms show. Though mumps is not highly contagious, a sufferer can infect others for about one week before the swelling and two weeks afterwards.

Symptoms and complications

Not all children become recognizably ill with mumps. Some are not susceptible, and others are immune because of a subclinical infection. Those who do become ill suffer in varying degree.

Some children might have a high fever and very swollen cheeks, while others might have no fever at all and only mild swelling. Where the pancreatic gland has been the main target of the infection, a child will vomit and have colicky pains. When a child has continuous, severe headaches and will not sit up in bed, the cerebral membrane is probably involved and the child has mumps meningitis. This condition is often not recognized, and there are usually no after-effects in children. It is often possible to avoid sending the child to hospital and nearly always possible to avoid a lumbar puncture. Antibiotic treatment in this case would be useless because the disease is caused by a viral infection.

If a boy or man gets mumps after puberty, there is a risk of getting an inflamed testicle, which is very painful and may cause the testicle to lose its function. In rare cases where both testicles are affected, infertility can result. While inflammation of the ovaries may also occur, it usually does not have any serious consequences.

Deafness after mumps only occurs in one in fifteen thousand cases, and true encephalitis occurs even more rarely, though all such statistics should be viewed with caution.

Treatment
For home treatment apply Archangelica Ointment (Weleda) or warm lavender-oil compresses to the swollen cheeks. For abdominal pain, use a damp compress with chamomile or yarrow infusion on the abdomen. In the latter case, the diet should be free of fats.

In general, high fever should not be brought down, but consult your doctor on this point. Fever weakens the activity of the virus and consequently tends to prevent possible complications.

WHOOPING COUGH (PERTUSSIS)

In the case of whooping cough, there is no automatic immunity through the mother, and all babies, even those who are breast-fed, are vulnerable. However, the question of immunization against whooping cough has been somewhat controversial in recent years.

Symptoms
After an incubation period of ten to fifteen days, the first sign of the illness is a harmless cough. This too lasts for ten to fifteen days before the child develops the characteristic "whoop" or crowing noise as he or she tries to draw breath. The whoop may continue for twenty to thirty days, so that the whole course of the illness from the first coughing to the final abatement can run four to six weeks.

In the first stage, known as the catarrhal stage, there is often a slight rise in temperature and the child is likely to have cold symptoms with a runny nose.

The next stage, with the characteristic whoop, is known as the paroxysmal (or spasmodic) stage. Mucus collects in the bronchial tubes, bringing on the loud, staccato cough that is an attempt to clear the mucus. The paroxysms wake the child during the night at intervals as frequent as every half-hour. After each cough, the child has trouble catching his or her breath, with the result that the face swells up and turns bluish. After some seconds, there comes the long, whooping in-breath through the constricted glottis. This is repeated once or twice. Finally the child coughs up the mucus, and possibly some recently eaten food, and falls asleep again, exhausted.

After each paroxysm, you can offer the child some liquid nourishment that will be absorbed by the gut before the next paroxysm starts.

The paroxysms themselves do not last longer than half a minute. It is important for parents to handle the situation calmly and gently. Slapping or thumping the child's back, or pulling the child up out of bed, will only make matters worse and will not help to ease the spasm. Younger children may simply lie on their stomachs, push themselves up, cough away, and then lie down again.

At the beginning of each bout, children feel very vulnerable. To help ease the breathing, talk them through the crisis calmly and encouragingly: "Cough it all up. Now breathe in and cough again. "This will help them to accept what is happening and not panic. Often the calm presence of an adult is enough, and so it is a good idea for one parent to spend the night in the same room with the child.

Fever at this stage is abnormal; if it develops, the doctor should be called immediately.

During the illness your child will lose weight, but do not worry. It is quite common for children to develop an extremely good appetite afterwards.

Exposure
Whooping cough is contagious from the start of the coughing until about four weeks later (in rare cases, six weeks). Whooping cough in babies less than three months old is a cause for concern, because at this young age babies cannot really manage the coughing fits and there is a high risk of complications. Therefore every precaution should be taken with young babies to avoid infection. Mothers with babies whose older brothers and sisters have not had whooping cough should be warned if there are cases in the area. The doctor can then, if the action is taken in time, arrest the infection in babies by giving an antibiotic.

Three- to six-month-old babies can still suffer the illness badly but are usually able to cope better with the coughing. Whooping cough in healthy babies over three months old has often been treated successfully without recourse to antibiotics. With proper treatment, complications are rare in children over one year old.

Treatment

Wrap the child up warmly in bed and give a hot linden tea so that the child sweats for a time. Then change the bed sheets and put the child into dry clothes, applying a lemon compress to the neck and throat or chest (see *Practical Home Care Medicine*, Lantern Books, 2001).

Sedatives and cough suppressants only increase the dangers of whooping cough in both babies and older children. These agents weaken the cough and reduce its frequency, allowing mucus to remain in the lungs. This can result in pneumonia and lack of oxygen to the brain. The illness can be more sensibly and less dangerously treated with medicines of anthroposophical and homeopathic origin. In the case of a delicate child with pneumonia, treatment with antibiotics can be considered. In normal cases, antibiotics can be used to stop the infection from spreading further, but they have no influence on the actual course of the illness, other than prevention if administered early enough.

Special Considerations

If a child has rickets or lacks calcium in his or her diet, whooping cough is much more dangerous. We always recommend that babies under one year of age with whooping cough be examined for this condition.

Babies admitted to the hospital make much better progress if their mothers are admitted with them.

Reprinted from *A Guide to Child Health* by permission of Floris Books, Edinburgh, 2002

❧ How to Treat Childhood Illnesses

Philip Incao, M.D.

"The best doctors are Dr. Diet, Dr. Quiet and Dr. Merryman."
—William Bullein

All of the common illnesses of childhood are inflammations. "Infection" is the wrong word for them, because it suggests that we get sick because germs invade us. This is misleading. We are always exposed to and often harbor germs, and yet we only occasionally get sick. Why do we get sick when we do?

In order to be healthy, we must keep an inner balance in body and soul while all the time growing and changing from birth to death. Childhood is the time of most rapid growth and dramatic change, and a child will remodel and renew his body many times as he grows. Every remodeling job requires some demolition, a breaking down of part of the inherited bodily structure in order to rebuild it better. This breaking down of old cells and tissues results in debris that must be cleaned up before the body rebuilds itself. It is the immune system that does the breaking down by causing cell death and, when necessary, fever and inflammation to destroy and digest foreign or outworn bodily material. And it is the immune system that cleans up the digested material and debris by pushing it out of the body. That is why children so often will have skin rashes and discharges of mucus or pus, *because their immune systems are actively working.* Debris that remains in the body may act like a poison, or may cause allergies or repeated inflammations later on. Germs do not "attack" us, but they often multiply wherever the body's living substance is dying, breaking down, and being discharged. Germs don't cause illnesses; they feed on them.

Every childhood inflammation, every cold, sore throat, earache, fever, and rash is a healing crisis and a cleansing process, a strong effort by the human spirit to remodel the body, to make it a more suitable dwelling. Anthroposophic and homeopathic remedies aid and promote this cleansing process and help the illness to work its way *out* of the body so that healing can occur. Antibiotics, aspirin, ibuprofen, and other anti-inflammatory drugs cool down and suppress the "fire" of the immune system so that the symptoms subside *before* the illness has fully worked its way out of the body. When an inflammation is suppressed in this way and prevented from fully discharging its toxins, then either the inflammation will come back, or else the tendency to allergies and asthma will be increased. Recent research has confirmed that antibiotics and vaccinations are a cause of increased allergies and asthma.

Although an antibiotic may be needed if the inflammatory response of the immune system gets out of control, this rarely happens in healthy people. Antibiotics never heal an inflammation; they only suppress it. The causes of the inflammation must still be healed after the antibiotic treatment; otherwise, the immune system may remain weakened.

Cleansing and Detox

In addition to any remedies you may use, *the first and best thing you should always do* at the onset of any inflammation, fever, cold, or "infection" is to cleanse the body as follows:

1. Give infants a glycerin rectal suppository. For adults and children over one year of age, give a bisacodyl (Dulcolax) suppository. If you prefer, an enema may be used instead of a suppository. (Of course, do not use any of these if diarrhea is present). *After the initial suppository or enema, it is important to keep the cleansing going until the illness is over by giving a dose of milk of magnesia once daily for three to five days*:

   Children 1–5 years of age: 1–2 tablespoons or 2–4 tablets
   Children 5–12 years of age: 2–3 tablespoons or 4–6 tablets
   Over 12 and adults: 4 tablespoons or 6–8 tablets

   After the first three to five days and until fever and pain are all gone, stewed prunes will help to keep the bowels loose.
   In infants under one year, fennel tea and diluted juices from stewed organic apricots and prunes will help to loosen the stools.

2. Drink lots of warm herb teas, especially horsetail (equisetum), which cleanses the kidneys.

3. *Strictly avoid all protein foods!* See "Diet" for further details.

Body Warmth and Fever

Children should always be warmly dressed for the weather. This will increase their bodies' ability to handle inflammations. The normal body temperature in a healthy child or adult should be 98.6 degrees or slightly higher, but preferably not lower. A subnormal temperature indicates that not enough warmth is being produced by the body. Viruses and bacteria grow faster and toxins accumulate when there is a lower-than-normal body temperature, and they are cleared faster from the body by the immune system when body temperature is higher. Weather permitting, young children should be dressed in natural fibers with three layers on top and two on the bottom. Wool socks will help support a healthy body temperature. Children under three years especially should wear caps or hats to protect the body from both warmth loss and the intensity of the sun.

Fever should not be regarded as a dangerous or unhealthy process in the body. It is actually a healthy response to the presence of something foreign or toxic that the body needs to get rid of. If we feel very uncomfortable, achy, or even delirious with fever, these are symptoms caused by the toxicity, the poisons, in our system. The fever isn't the problem; it's part of the solution! Giving acetaminophen or ibuprofen for a fever is like killing the messenger.

Many parents have a dread of fevers because they expect them to lead to convulsions or brain damage. These fears are unnecessary. The great majority of fevers are perfectly benign, and the great majority of children are not susceptible to fever convulsions and don't get them with even very high fevers. Fever convulsions happen only in a small minority of children who are so constituted as to have a low threshold for convulsions. Even in these susceptible children, fever convulsions are rare events, usually happening only once or twice between six months and six years of age. Keep in mind that:

- Fever convulsions do not cause any permanent damage to the brain or nervous system.
- Lowering a fever with medications, baths, or anything else will *not* prevent convulsions, and it is best to avoid these methods. In fact, recent research suggests that *fever-lowering drugs may actually harm the patient* by suppressing the immune system and increasing the body's retention of toxicity, thus making complications and prolongation of the illness more likely.
- The minority of children who are susceptible to fever convulsions will outgrow their susceptibility after age 7.
- *A fever convulsion is much less likely to occur* if the recommendations in these pages for bowel cleansing, diet, quiet, and warmth are promptly followed at the first sign of illness in children, and the appropriate anthroposophic or homeopathic remedies are given.

It is the *toxicity* from certain diseases and certain immunizations that may in rare instances cause brain damage or convulsions in children or adults, regardless of whether the fever is high or low. But fever by itself, even when it reaches 104 degrees or over, will not cause brain damage. In the very rare case when a fever goes over 106 degrees, you should call your doctor.

When your child has a fever, dress him or her even *more warmly* than usual in layers of cotton or wool. Keep the patient warm enough that the cheeks are red and the hands and feet are warm, but there is no sweat or perspiration. The body in its wisdom wants and needs to be hot in order to burn out the illness. When the fever is rising, we feel chilled and want to get warm under blankets. When the fever breaks and then starts to come down, only then do we feel hot and sweat and throw off the blankets. This is the natural way the immune system burns out the illness and discharges its toxins.

Since fever drives the toxins out of the body, fever-reducing drugs can make us more toxic! This explains why, in some viral inflammations of children, aspirin increases the risk of Reye's syndrome, and ibuprofen and possibly acetaminophen may increase the risk of serious bacterial complications. Acetaminophen has a well-known toxic effect on the liver that can be very dangerous at higher doses. It may also increase the tendency to asthma, which is a rapidly growing problem in today's children.

Healing occurs when our toxins have been fully digested and discharged from the body. Traditional medical wisdom has always recognized that the pus discharge, mucus, or rash is a *healing response* to the underlying illness.

If a child or adult with a high fever is very uncomfortable and restless, this is a sign of toxicity and the previously mentioned cleansing measures are needed. You may also rub the arms, legs, and head with a washcloth moistened with tepid water and Arnica tincture or lemon juice. (From the neck to the knees the child should not be undressed.) Rub vigorously to make the skin red; this will help to dissipate excess body heat through the skin. Restlessness and irritability during a fever are caused by circulating toxins in the body and can often be prevented by following the directions under "Cleansing and Detox."

Diet
When someone has or is coming down with any type of inflammation, cold, or fever, the diet should be restricted. When your

body is trying to "digest" and eliminate toxic substances it will help if you don't have to digest much food at the same time. Therefore, the general rule is to *avoid protein foods* during the acute illness. These include meat, eggs, dairy, nuts, fish, and legumes (beans, peas, lentils, soy, etc.).

The sick person should have a mainly liquid diet of vegetable broth, herb teas, and fruit juices, but no juices colder than room temperature. Fruit, cooked vegetables, grains, and light crackers are also suitable.

Another general rule is that when sick, eating *less* is better than eating more. If the patient is not hungry, she is better off not eating. On the other hand, when your patient in the middle of her illness is suddenly hungry, feed her light, nonprotein food and she will be quickly satisfied. Add protein only when you are *sure* the illness is really over.

The return of appetite is a sign of getting over the illness, but those first meals after the fever is gone should be light ones. Don't be too eager to have your child regain lost weight; this will happen soon enough quite naturally as your child's appetite and strength return. After the illness, reintroduce the restricted foods gradually and carefully.

Quiet

During a fever or any inflammatory illness, we crave peace and quiet and are disturbed by noises and sounds that usually don't bother us when we are well. Children need peace and quiet during their illnesses, though they will rarely express this need. Instead, out of "boredom" they will ask to listen to the radio or tapes, or to watch TV. These kinds of stimulation are best avoided, especially in younger children, and should be replaced by just "being there" for your child during his or her illness in a peaceful, unhurried, and reassuring way. Keep sick children quietly under the covers in bed or on a couch away from the hustle and bustle of household activity. The more they can sleep during an illness, the better.

Illness is a time to remove oneself from the usual pressures and routines of life, to "veg out" totally and to allow one's body to repair and renew itself in the context of a peaceful and supportive environment. Very often illness can provide a wonderful opportunity for renewed communication and bonding between parent and child.

Dr. Merryman: Mastering Fear

The cleansing and detox and other recommendations in these pages have proven themselves to work extremely well in over eighty years of experience with anthroposophic medicine in many countries of the world. They have worked extremely well for my patients, including my own three children, since I began practicing medicine in 1972.

Pediatric medical journals have addressed the phenomenon of "fever phobia," the unreasoning and unwarranted fear of fever that many parents have. Fear is a natural response to the experience of powerful forces we do not understand. Acute inflammation and fever are certainly poorly understood, powerful forces; nevertheless they are *healing* forces!

When fear gains the upper hand, clear vision and judgment go out the window. If we can master our fear and sit calmly and reassuringly with our children when they are ill, observing them carefully, there is much we can learn. We may find that our fear gives way to a healthy respect and a glimmer of understanding for the change emerging in our child through the ebb and flow of the fever.

In every fever and inflammation, forces of body, soul, and spirit are working to bring to birth a new order and a new balance. Many mothers have told me of their child's developmental leap in emotional and neurological maturity after working through a feverish illness. That's because every fever and inflammation is like a labor pain in childbirth. They're not pleasant, but just as labor pains help the child's body to come out into the world, so do fevers and inflammations help the child's spirit and soul come out into the world. This "coming out" of the child's spirit and soul is a stepwise process that enables the child to master and control his or her own body and to relate to his or her environment—the very same miraculous process that is responsible for the child's healthy growth and development. This process is what feverish illnesses support and enhance in children, provided that these illnesses are able to run their course in a healthy way, and to accomplish their important work of remodeling and renewing the human body.

Every mother knows how helpful it is during labor and childbirth to be surrounded by loving people who create a warm, supportive, and positive atmosphere. A child laboring through his or her feverish illness needs just this kind of loving, positive support from the adults who are the midwives in this birth process of the child's spirit and soul.

If we could learn to greet fever in ourselves or our children as the special event that it is, and as a sign that the new balance and the fresh start we needed is now coming about, imagine the difference such an attitude would make! Instead of regarding a cold, flu, or fever as an unwelcome interruption in our life and feeling worried, anxious, or annoyed, we might realize with awe and respect that the deeper wisdom we needed is now actively working through us or our children. Such a positive attitude helps greatly to bring about a healthy outcome.

Of course, as with any birth process, we need to be observant and discerning to make sure the inflammation unfolds in a healthy way and to know when to call for expert help. This knowledge and judgment can be gained through experience, so that with each illness in our children we become more familiar with the inflammatory process and more sure of our ability to judge its healthy limits.

Often, children themselves have an intuitive understanding of what they are experiencing as they work through a feverish inflammatory illness, and occasionally they express it. One five-year-old patient of mine said to his concerned mother at the peak of his illness, "Don't worry Mom, I'm just growing!"

All growing requires that the ground first be broken and made fertile. That is what feverish inflammatory illnesses do for us and our children.

Reprinted from *Lilipoh* #24, 2001

✎ Creating a Healing Environment

Mary Kelly Sutton, M.D.

A sense of mystery exists around illness. We tend to ask, "Why me?" or "Why now?" and "Why this particular illness?" We know from experience the impact illness has on our lives. Often after an illness a child will take a developmental step forward. So illness is a means for transformation.

When creating a healing environment in the home, we want to make space for both the practical and the mysterious to work themselves out.

Looking at the Individual

The first step for the caregiver is to take a good look at the sick individual. A calm, receptive tone will create the right environment for the sick person to express his or her needs. Sometimes sickness brings over-sensitivity and a demanding mood. The caregiver should try to recognize this as part of the illness and not take it personally. Quiet talk with a child suffering from chicken pox, recalling our own chicken pox miseries, lets the sick one hear someone else's struggle put into words. The child will feel relief at being understood. When the caregiver respects the sick person's dignity and has faith in the recovery, then the caregiver becomes like a medicine to the patient. A sick child doesn't care about remedies, but just wants the presence of the loving parent. As the process unfolds, the sick person's sense of self changes from vulnerability to a new independence.

A quiet environment contributes to healing, and so TV and technically produced sounds have little place in creating a healing space. Sleep should be protected—even the administering of remedies should be avoided if the child is in a sound sleep.

All the recommendations here and below are to be individualized for the sick child. But remember that this discussion should be treated as a source of questions to be asked rather than predetermined answers. The answer is in the patient.

Rhythm

The body follows precise and timely rhythms in secreting hormones and enzymes in synchronicity with the changing times of day or year around us. We gain much more security and support from a meal or a remedy when our treatments are given with regularity.

For growing children, rhythm in life provides a strong foundation in their physiology, so that as adults, when schedules are erratic, their body function is secure from years of rhythmic living. For the sick adult, use of rhythm is a return to that healthful time of childhood, and brings health more quickly to the sufferer.

Cleansing

The physical effect of an illness is to bring about a body cleansing that is fundamental to healing. If we cooperate with that effort, the body can finish its work quickly and effectively.

At the onset of illness, inflammation, or fever, a sick person should be helped to empty the bowels thoroughly, first with an enema, if the patient is comfortable with this, or with a Dulcolax (bisacodyl) suppository (the adult size can be used beginning at the age of one year). The bowel cleansing should be continued for several days and followed by milk of magnesia, Smoothe Move tea, Laxadoron tablets (Weleda), prunes, or whatever works for that person. The goal is to have one more than the usual number of bowel movements per day.

Whether as plain water or as a carrier for an herb or oil, fluids carry healing properties. A warm mist vaporizer with eucalyptus oil assists relief of congestion in almost all respiratory conditions. Inhalation (with chamomile, or chamomile and eucalyptus) produces a concentrated humidity for quick relief of mucus and soothing of irritated passages. Because asthma may become worse with concentrated humidity or odors, it is important to use caution in asthmatic patients.

Hot lemonade (honey, fresh lemon, and hot water), miso soup, vegetable broth (no monosodium glutamate, please), and herb teas can be drunk warm to hot in large quantities (up to two gallons per day). Urinary output is an important measure of hydration, and when a person has no urine output for twelve hours, or has significantly diminished urine output in the presence of fever, it is imperative that the doctor be notified quickly.

Warmth

Warmth is of such prime importance in healing that it stands alone. Lack of warmth underlies chronic illness more often than we realize. The addition of warmth maintains health in a well person, and supports healing in a sick one.

Warmth exists on many levels. The body creates physical warmth in the form of fever in an effort to rouse the immune system to action and bring the illness process to completion. The presence of fever is the signal of a competent immune system, and of the action of the organizing forces of the sick person trying to take charge. Fever has been known to cure illnesses, including some cancers, and some current research is based on these findings.

Emotional warmth is the foundation of children's total growth, and, though not quite as critical to adult survival, it is essential for adult well-being. Sincere interest in the sick person and willingness to listen and grow in understanding of his or her particular situation and makeup are the caregiver's gifts of warmth to the patient. They may be delivered with objectivity, as by a health professional, or with great attachment, as by a parent. But in either case, the support of companionship and human warmth during illness promotes healing.

Reprinted from *Lilipoh* #2, 1995, from the *Home Care Course* given by Mary Kelly Sutton and Thomas Cowan, M.D.

A Safe and Natural Approach to Childhood Illnesses

Wiep de Vries, R.N.

Parents and caretakers are generally uncomfortable dealing with children's illnesses. Illness brings up feelings of worry and fear that something has gone wrong, as if the body is breaking down. Yet illness is part of who we are. Illness holds within itself invisible intentionality and has a "language" of its own. It plays a crucial role in a child's development and manifests itself in the form of symptoms coming into expression as the whole body sets out on a path to find a renewed balance, a higher level of integration and consolidation. Rudolf Steiner explains that illness points toward something in our future; it is a mirror image of what a person needs to accomplish.

Our Self-Healing Nature
A child's intricate process of change and renewal is best served when parents and caretakers can support and nurture the sick child from a place of compassion while having the practical tools to carefully guide the child through his or her challenges. In overcoming *dis-ease*, a child goes through an important learning process that involves body, soul, and spirit.

In Europe many doctors choose to let illnesses run their course, since studies show that antibiotics often do not affect the progress and duration of an illness. The current medical approach in the U.S. is to prescribe suppressive medicine, such as antibiotics and vaccinations, thereby inhibiting the process of individualization.

I have found that once parents have learned what they can expect during a childhood illness, their dependence on health care services is much less. The challenge is to go beyond the fear and develop insights and tools to support your child in times of illness. A sick child craves your undivided attention and nurturing and will respond energetically to your state of mind, whether it is one of fear or of support. Realizing that children's self-healing abilities are very powerful, we choose to carefully guide and support the child through the process of illness. Voltaire said about two hundred years ago, "The art of medicine consists of amusing the patient while nature cures the disease." Edgar Cayce indicated that the body's innate healing ability is the direct result of the manifestation of Spirit within it. "For, all healing must come from the Divine. Healing requires the 'attuning of each atom'—no matter what we do for our health—it is to bring the consciousness of creative or God forces."

Our Inner Warmth
Long-term stress and suppression of fever can harm a child's natural ability to bring forth the dynamic changes in internal warmth. All diseases start with a change in the warmth of body and soul. This may be better understood when we learn to see how the processes of warmth are the highest expression of our spirit activity. Our inner warmth provides a means for our spirit to be engaged in our bodies.

I feel that care for the warmth organization of the child is the immediate task of parents and caregivers, because the energy of the redirecting and reorganizing forces of our higher self is based in the warmth of the blood.

Warmth comes from our spirit and is transferred to the soul, where it lives as soul warmth—sympathy, true interest, love, and compassion. Only in a warm inner environment can transformation take place. Warmth stands at the beginning of every creation, serving the process of becoming.

Basic Guidelines for Caring for a Child with Fever

A child with a fever goes through a profound learning process as the warmth penetrates deeply into the body to activate a metabolic response. The metabolic activity generates an inner fire, which is the impulse for the renewal of the body. It is the inner fire that activates the cellular immune system into the mode of discharge and elimination of toxic matter. After the phase of elimination the child starts to rebuild his or her own body proteins. All our interventions are geared toward assisting the fever and encouraging elimination and discharge. Following such principles results in a smooth and quick recovery. A key element in this process is having a caregiver you can work with, who also understands these principles and will support and comfort you.

Aspects of Care

- Dress your child in several layers and avoid any temperature fluctuations, since this will take energy away from the healing process. Feel your child's hands, feet, and belly. Areas of coldness require a hot water bottle. As a rule, we keep the head cool and the extremities and the abdomen warm to allow the fever to do its job quietly and smoothly—always taking care that the child remains comfortable. Don't "over-warm"!

- Avoid baths when a fever is developing or present, because the child can easily become chilled. All the body's warmth is needed for healing.

- When there is no fever present, a fifteen-minute herbal sweat bath with eucalyptus bath salts in it can speed healing. Afterwards, immediately wrap the child in fresh clothes and bedclothes, and give a pleasant warm drink.

- Try to avoid anti-inflammatory and fever-reducing medicines. These can inhibit the outbreak of rashes in diseases such as chicken pox and measles. When this happens, the illness can actually turn inwards and worsen or become prolonged. These days it is not uncommon to hear that children have a repetition of chicken pox. This is our bodily wisdom showing us that we need to help bring out an illness rather than suppress it. Investigate ways to support your child with herbal, homeopathic, or anthroposophical remedies.

- Your sick child is calling you to support his or her inner warmth with warming and nurturing love from your heart. This heartfelt connection between the parents or caretakers and the child is indispensable for a sense of safety, comfort, and peace.

- Avoid over-stimulation, such as exposure to noises, radio, and television. These can irritate the nervous system and deprive the child of much-needed rest.

- The sick child benefits from a calming and tidy environment with soft colors. The bed sheets and clothing should consist of natural fabrics.

- Allow your child additional time to fully recuperate.

When the Fever Gets Very Uncomfortable

- Close the curtains and avoid excess noise and movement in the room.
- Don't bathe the child at this time.
- Rub the lower arms and lower legs and neck several times with a rough washcloth moistened with tepid lemon water and/or diluted Arnica Essence.
- Make lemon calf socks to draw the inflammation down from the head area.

Cleansing

Unless a child has diarrhea, you can immediately help to relieve his or her symptoms by promoting internal cleansing. Give a mild laxative, like milk of magnesia, or a glycerin suppository for two to three days to promote detoxification. Fennel tea is great for infants under one year of age.

Often, an enema with warm catnip tea or chamomile tea will help make the child more comfortable.

Dosage for milk of magnesia once daily for three to five days is as follows:

Children 1–5 years of age: 1–2 tablespoons or 2–4 tablets
Children 5–10 years of age: 2–3 tablespoons or 4–6 tablets
Over 10 and adults: 3–4 tablespoons or 6–8 tablets

Congestion and Cough

- Use a hot steam vaporizer with eucalyptus oil.
- Rub Weleda Archangelica/Eucalyptus Ointment on chest and back.
- Use hot teas, like Weleda Sytra Tea or chamomile tea.

Vomiting or Diarrhea

- Offer several teaspoons of chamomile tea every fifteen minutes. Mix in one teaspoon of an unflavored oral electrolyte solution if you worry about dehydration.
- Slowly introduce light foods as instructed in the nutrition section below.

Rash Care

Try these remedies for itching:

- Bath with oatmeal (Aveeno) or cornstarch once a day (if the fever is high, give sponge baths only)
- Sponge bath with tea made of goldenseal and burdock root
- Aloe vera gel, Combudoron gel, or calamine lotion

For Strengthening after the Illness

- Weleda Elixirs
- Prunus bath

Rhythm

The self-healing forces are most strongly addressed when the care is orchestrated in a flowing, rhythmical fashion. Structure any caring intervention, whether it is providing a meal or giving remedies, in a way that provides security, balance, and relaxation. It is important to be sensitive to this need for rhythm when your child is not well. You can consider such an approach as a medicine that brings harmony to the whole body.

Sleep

Sleep is the ultimate healer: during sleep the body builds itself up. At times of imbalance, the natural rhythms of life need maximum support to stimulate the child's self-healing and harmonizing forces. Providing a calming and loving environment helps promote the quality of sleep.

Basic Nutritional Guidelines

Avoid cold drinks. Serve warm fluids, such as vegetable broth or miso soup, hot lemonade with honey, chamomile tea, or elder flower tea.

The diet should be adjusted to light foods, such as grains, cream of rice, rice crackers, cooked vegetables, and vegetable broth. The body goes through a phase of breakdown and elimination and should not be burdened with the digestion of heavy proteins and fats, including meat, eggs, dairy, nuts, fish and legumes (beans, peas, lentils, soy). When the child's appetite comes back, gradually reintroduce proteins and fats in the meals.

★ ★ ★

For remedies to support a child through a childhood illness, as well as information about some of the treatments listed above, I recommend you refer to the book *Practical Home Care Medicine* (Lantern Books, 2001), which contains simple remedies and practical applications that you can use in conjunction with your physician's advice.

Part III

Treating the Effects of Immunization

An Anthroposophic View of the Immune System

William Warnock, N.D.

The immune system is the method by which the uniqueness of the individual's physical body is maintained so that it can be a truly worthy vessel for the ego. Immunizations at an early age interfere with this process. According to the Merck Manual, cell-mediated immunity does not reach maturity until about one year, and immunoglobulin levels are reached approximately as follows: IgM by one year, IgG by eight years, and IgA by eleven years. When immunization forces an accelerated maturation of the immune system by introducing such a large amount of antigen at once, the immune system loses the ability to complete its ideal development. In the same way, a person can walk on a new sidewalk before it completely hardens, but as a consequence the sidewalk remains forever blemished. While our powers of recuperation are great and the body is adaptable, a child goes through developmental stages that, once past, cannot be recaptured.

Because the child's etheric body (vital force) provides the energy for an immune response, his or her strong etheric ties with the mother and other caregivers are important. During gestation the unborn child experiences everything the mother experiences to the degree that physically and etherically they are one. Once the physical body is freed from the mother at birth, the child strives to overcome the residue of the mother's physical body. This process takes about seven years. The etheric body of the child during the first seven years is still strongly linked to the mother and, to a lesser degree, to the father or other caregiver. The degree of linkage depends on the individual situation. If the mother or other caregiver is under stress, this will affect the child. She or he will not be able to find the resources to mount an appropriate immune response to an immunization or to an illness.

Mother's milk contains antibodies and other immune-modulating substances and is the best counter-measure to the side effects of immunization. When a mother shares her milk with a baby, she shares a very intimate part of herself. Her milk has within it an abundance of physical and etheric forces that the baby can easily make use of, but these physical and etheric forces also contain residues of the mother's physical and emotional life. It is therefore essential that the mother take care of herself when she is nursing; proper nutrition, enough sleep, and calm emotions are all important. In anthroposophical medicine we know that because of the strong imprint of the mother on her milk, nursing has a tendency to slow down the child's own striving for independence. Vaccinations have the opposite effect, i.e., they speed up a child's development. Mother's milk therefore becomes a medicine given in response to immunization, and I recommend that a child who receives immunizations nurse longer than one who doesn't.

In general, the healthier a child is, the less he or she will suffer ill effects from the immunization. Also make sure the child (at whatever age) is getting enough sleep, a good diet, and plenty of water. Since immunizations have a cooling effect on a child's warmth ether, warmth is an essential hygienic component in counteracting immunizations, as long as it is not overdone. Solum Uliginosum Oil massaged into the abdomen and thighs each day can help stimulate the warmth organism.

Homeopathic remedies can be given to treat the acute effects of immunization. Consult your physician.

✎ Treating the Effects of Immunization

Mary Kelly Sutton, M.D.

A variety of supportive measures can be of value around the time of immunization. The topics of warmth and rhythm are each worthy of their own treatise. These non-bottled treatments are more fundamental than any herb or antibiotic or injection. It is in the use of these principles that we find the balance that gives the immune system its greatest strength, and the individual his or her fullest growth and expression. Whether we are handling a disease or a vaccination, the basic principles of warmth and rhythm are a foundation stone for health that we must not overlook, in spite of our busy lives. The day of a vaccination, and the next several days, should ideally be a bit monotonous (from an adult's point of view), as they provide a routine without additional exhaustion or stress for the immunized child.

One application of the principle of warmth is used by European pediatricians, who instruct parents to briskly rub children's calves with a terry cloth when the child has measles or another rash-producing disease. Bringing a pink color to the surface by this mild irritation improves circulation and draws the rash (inflammation) process outward to the skin, and downward to the limbs. What simple genius! The body wants to inflame and we direct it to do so at a safe location. The old saying, "the skin is the proper place for disease to happen" is exemplified by this treatment. The Harrison's textbook I used in medical school noted that chicken pox encephalitis commonly occurred with presence of very few pox. The body had directed the inflammation process deep into the organs instead of to the skin. Had this observation been developed, might we be warming our children instead of vaccinating them?

The knowledge is there for us to use, even if it is not common practice. The warm child (or adult) is the child with an immune system able to work safely. No longer is an acute illness a terrorist we might fear. We simply learn to manage it, with warmth, rest, cleansing, and some nontoxic natural substances that support the immune system in its work. This knowledge about warmth is so important that I include sources for wool underwear and headwear in the folder for newborns and ask adults to shop for their own layer of protection.

Following the practice of several anthroposophical physicians, I use Thuja 6X (Weleda) twice daily two weeks before and two weeks after each immunization as support for the immune work required by the immunization. I do not delay the immunization if someone has not begun Thuja ahead of time but simply use it three to four times daily afterward. Screening questions diminish the likelihood of vaccine reactions. When biorhythms and other physiological parameters are better understood by basic science, we will be able to time immunizations for the best effect.

❧ A Homeopathic Antidote for Vaccine-Related Illness

Rosemary Rau-Levine, M.D.

H er Serene Highness, Princess Antoinette of Monaco, is an animal lover. A few years ago, she decided to give an international conference for doctors, and invited Dr. Paul Nogier to present. In thirty years of research, Dr. Nogier, who invented ear acupuncture in the 1950s, used no animal subjects—only humans.

Dr. Nogier in turn invited the famous researcher Dr. Jacques Benveniste, who was known to have turned down the Ministry of Health for France to pursue his research work. Dr. Benveniste had proved that homeopathy could produce a reaction past the point where any of the original substance remained in the body. His research was published in the journal *Nature*. But his critics rushed to discredit him. After they hired a magician to announce that Benveniste's research was just like magic tricks—hocus pocus—*Nature* rescinded the article!

A young doctor presenting some new Benveniste research at the Monaco conference was so angry as he related the incident that he could hardly speak. He quieted himself and told us that the main intent of Benveniste's research was to prove that homeopathy works.

91

Benveniste's findings were as follows: When a rat was given a single homeopathic dose of metal daily for five days, then given a toxic dose of that same metal, fatal to unprepared rats, the rat's body could excrete seventy-five percent of the metal in the first twenty-four hours. With another dose of the homeopathic metal given one month later, the rat could excrete the last twenty-five percent of the metal and remain unharmed.

I was musing about how Princess Antoinette might have preferred this research to have been done, somehow, on humans instead of on rats, and in the darkened auditorium in Monaco, surrounded by doctors from all over the world, I thought of the many mothers who ask me to get vaccination substances out of their children's bodies after the antibodies have been formed. If there was an ongoing human counterpart to Benveniste's research, this was it, except that the children had not received the homeopathic vaccine five days in advance.

The moms at home pose this question to me because the illnesses they noted in their children one to two weeks after their vaccinations have become chronic by the time they consult me, years later, in my office.

I had started a laboratory to make homeopathic remedies, and decided to replicate Benveniste's findings. But how would I know if the vaccine substance had been excreted? Then a family contacted our lab. Could we get lead out of their child's body? She had been exposed to old lead paint in their Victorian house, and had a high blood lead level.

Here was a chance to see if, retrospectively, we could remove lead by homeopathic means. And indeed, the blood lead level came to "below normal" levels after the homeopathic protocol.

After that, we prospectively used the protocol to get radioactive iodine out of a woman's body in twenty-four hours. She was to be injected with it to test for thyroid cancer. The doctor who checked her with his Geiger counter afterwards couldn't believe it; he thought the batteries must be dead.

Because of the above instances and others like them, I saw that the homeopathic protocol could work to remove vaccines and other substances from my patients. The moms have been using the prevaccination kits since 1990 with good results. The mercury/dental kits work, too.

I think Her Serene Highness, Princess of Monaco, would be pleased.

Reprinted from *Lilipoh* #24, 2001

Note: Celletech (see Resources) produces the pre-vaccination, post-vaccination, and heavy metal detoxification protocols discussed by Dr. Rau-Levine. In collaboration over nineteen years, Dr. Rau-Levine and John Cain developed these and other protocols based on the research of Drs. Jacques Benveniste and Sigrun Seutemann.

⚈ Summary

Philip Incao, M.D.

E veryone experiences acute inflammations. Colds, the flu, and fevers, seem to be an inescapable part of life. Why do we get them? Many of us have noticed (if not, then our spouses have noticed!) that we often come down with a cold or flu when we are overly stressed or depleted. We explain this by assuming that stress lowers our resistance to the viruses and bacteria that, we believe, like to attack us and make us sick. In fact, most of the time we peacefully coexist with these microbes that share our environment; if we get sick, it's often because we've allowed ourselves to get out of balance. This applies to children too, but imbalance is not the only cause of childhood illness.

Studies have shown that in children, respiratory infections increase in frequency from birth until a peak by age six, followed by a sharp decline after age seven, irrespective of treatment. In other words, it seems to be a normal feature of childhood to experience a variety of acute inflammations, especially respiratory illnesses, in the first seven years of life.

Prior to the advent of twentieth-century improvements in sanitation and living standards, children had a high death rate in their first seven years from these acute inflammations: measles, scarlet fever, diphtheria, whooping cough, and the common unnamed pneumonias and diarrheas. These have been the greatest threats to children throughout history, and in developing countries, they still are. In all modern nations, however, children's deaths from such acute inflammations have been steeply declining ever since 1900, and over ninety percent of the decline occurred before the advent of antibiotics and vaccinations.[1]

In the U.S. today, what used to be the common dangerous infections of childhood account for only about one percent of children's deaths. (In contrast, seven percent of deaths in American children ages one to nineteen are from cancer, seven percent are from suicide, and a shocking fourteen percent are from homicide.) Now, growing numbers of children are living with chronic disease: for example, since 1960 there has been a sharp increase in both the frequency and the severity of asthma in many developed nations. In the U.S., asthma accounts for one percent of children's deaths—equal to infections—and is a leading cause of childhood disability.

A growing body of medical research supports the commonsense idea that otherwise healthy children who experience frequent infections and inflammations in early childhood will strengthen their immune systems and will be less prone to allergies and asthma than children who rarely experience such infections. This idea is called "the hygiene hypothesis." Research has revealed a list of factors (see below) that correlate with a decreased risk of asthma and allergies, including the avoidance of vaccinations and antibiotics.

If the hygiene hypothesis proves to be correct, it will have a revolutionary impact on medical practice. We will realize that, when children experience their colds and fevers, they are challenging their immune systems and developing an inner strength that will be theirs to draw on throughout life. As with all chal-

---

Factors correlating with lower risk of allergies and asthma[2]

- Having older siblings
- Entering daycare by six months old
- Reacting positive to a TB skin test
- Having had the measles
- Not having had the DPT or MMR vaccinations
- Having had little or no antibiotics, especially before the age of two
- Eating fermented foods containing live lactobacilli
- Growing up with frequent exposure to farm animals
- Not washing much

---

lenges in childhood, our job as parents and health care workers will be to strengthen the child to meet his or her challenges by not removing the challenges altogether. In the long run, it's not possible to eliminate challenges, but only to replace some kinds of challenges with other kinds.

The blessing of modern medicine is that it has the tools and techniques to ease suffering and save lives when we or our children are in danger of being overwhelmed by illness.

Nevertheless, thwarting or suppressing illness does not automatically create health, although it can be quite justified in an acute or life-threatening situation, granting the body enough respite to be able to start the healing process. Health and healing are mostly about developing our inner capacities to adapt to change and to maintain balance as we move through life's journey.

To truly foster the overall health and inner strength of our children, we need to go beyond the short-sighted view of illnesses as hostile aggressors and of children as helpless victims. Children are individuals. Each child gets ill in his or her own individual way, and each illness a child gets has a meaningful part to play among the challenges belonging to that child's life. Just like everything else in nature, individual illnesses exist within a larger context of a balanced system. There is an ecology of human illness. If we attempt to eliminate a single element of an ecological system, we disturb the balance of the whole in ways that can lead to unforeseen consequences.

To these unforeseen consequences belong the dramatic increases in asthma, allergies, diabetes, autism, and learning dysfunctions occurring in children today. These result, in part, from modern medicine's failure to appreciate where the balance lies in health and illness, and from its failure to grasp that when you push down on one side of the balance, the other side goes up! Our present effort to eradicate acute infectious diseases in children through increasing numbers of vaccines has already long overshot the healthy balance point, and is now helping to create in developed nations more chronic disease and disability in children than ever before.

To improve public health, policy needs to shift its focus from eradicating particular diseases to improving the social conditions that breed disease, and physicians need to learn how to help our individual patients to maintain balance in body, soul, and spirit throughout their lives. If we physicians learn that, and if we apply it to ourselves as well, then the overall health of our society cannot help but improve.

1. Polio is an important exception to this pattern, resembling the modern degenerative illnesses more closely than the classical inflammatory illnesses. Just before 1900, when all the other familiar life-threatening children's illnesses were beginning to decline, the newcomer polio made its first appearance in medical history and continued to grow in importance until its abrupt decline with the advent of the Salk and Sabin polio vaccines in the 1950s.

2. Based on the following references:

Alm J. S., Swartz J., Lilja G., Scheynius A., Pershagen G. "Atopy in children of families with an anthroposophic lifestyle." *Lancet* 353 (1999): 1485–88.

Ball T. M., Castro-Rodriguez J. A., Griffith K. A., Holberg C. J., Martinez F .D., Wright A. L. "Siblings, day-care attendance, and the risk of asthma and wheezing during childhood." *The New England Journal of Medicine* 343 (2002): 538–43.

Bodner C., Anderson W. J., Reid T. S., Godden D. J. "Childhood exposure to infection and risk of adult onset wheeze and atopy." *Thorax* 55, no. 5 (2000): 383–7.

Hurwitz E. L., Morgenstern H. "Effects of Diphtheria-Tetanus-Pertussis or Tetanus vaccination on allergies and allergy-related respiratory symptoms among children and adolescents in the United States." *Journal of Manipulative and Physiological Therapeutics* 23, no. 2 (2000): 81–89.

Kramer U., Heinrich J., Wjst M., Wichmann H. E. "Age of entry to day nursery and allergy in later childhood." *Lancet* 352 (1998): 450–54.

Ponsonby A. L., Couper D., Dwyer T., Carmichael A. "Cross sectional study of the relation between sibling numbers and asthma, hay fever, and eczema." *Archives of Disease in Childhood* 79 (1998): 328–33.

Riedler J., et al. *Clinical and Experimental Allergy*, Dec. 1999.

Rona R. J., Duran-Tauleria E., Chinn S. "Family size, atopic disorders in parents, asthma in children, and ethnicity." *The Journal of Allergy and Clinical Immunology* 99 (1997): 454–60.

Shaheen S. O., Aaby P., Hall A. J., Barker D. J. P., et al. "Measles and atopy in Guinea-Bissau." *Lancet* 347 (1996): 1792–1796.

Strachan D. P., Harkins L. S., Johnston I. D. A., Anderson H. R. "Childhood antecedents of allergic sensitization in young British adults." *The Journal of Allergy and Clinical Immunology* 99 (1997): 6–T2.

Strachan D. P., Taylor E. M., Carpenter R. G. "Family structure, neonatal infection, and hay fever in adolescence." *Archives of Disease in Childhood* 74 (1996): 422–6.

Strachan D. P. "Hayfever, hygiene, and household size." *BMJ* 299 (1989): 1259–60.

Von Mutius E., Martinez F. D., Fritzsch C., Nicolai T., Reitmer P., Thiemann H. H. "Skin test reactivity and number of siblings." *BMJ* 308 (1994): 692–5.

∞ Contributors

Wiep de Vries, R.N. is a registered nurse and massage therapist who has worked in an anthroposophical hospital in the Netherlands. She currently teaches holistic home health care programs for parents and caregivers in the greater Los Angeles area. She is the founder of the Los Angeles Alliance for Childhood, a multidisciplinary family support network.

Barbara Loe Fisher is co-author of *DPT: A Shot in the Dark* and co-founder and president of the National Vaccine Information Center in Vienna, Virginia, a non-profit educational organization founded in 1982. In 1999 she was appointed as the consumer voting member of the FDA Vaccines and Related Biological Products Advisory Committee, where she will serve until 2003.

Michaela Gloeckler, M.D. spent many years practicing pediatric medicine at the Community Hospital in Herdeke, Germany and as a Waldorf School physician. In 1988 she was appointed Head of the Medical Section of the Goetheanum in Dornach, Switzerland, and since then has represented the anthroposophical approach to health worldwide.

Wolfgang Goebel, M.D. co-founded the Community Hospital in Herdeke, Germany, where he also directed the children's wing for many years. Dr. Goebel has been active as a school physician in Waldorf Schools. The book *A Guide to Child Health*, co-authored with Dr. Gloeckler, establishes the connection between education and healing.

Philip Incao, M.D. has practiced family medicine for over twenty-five years and is one of only a handful of American physicians who practice anthroposophic medicine. Dr. Incao has studied vaccinations and their effects first-hand and has lectured and written extensively on the topic. He has a medical practice in Denver and Boulder, Colorado.

Rosemary Rau-Levine, M.D. has been in practice for thirty-seven years, specializing in family alternative medicine since 1979. She is certified in anthroposophical medicine, homeopathy, body and ear acupuncture, cranial manipulation, and child, adolescent, and adult psychiatry. She is also an art therapist. Dr. Rau-Levine lives in San Francisco, California.

Mary Kelly Sutton, M.D. is a founding member of the American Holistic Medical Association and has worked as a primary care physician in the U.S. and in the Middle East since 1971. In 1991 she received Boards from the American College of Anthroposophically Extended Medicine. She now practices in Keene, New Hampshire.

William Warnock, N.D. (naturopathic doctor) has been in practice since 1984. He uses anthroposophical, herbal, and homeopathic treatments for children's developmental issues and illnesses. He also helps people in the treatment of many chronic diseases such as cancer, diabetes, Chronic Fatigue and Immune Dysfunction Syndrome (CFIDS), and fibromyalgia. He is the founder of the Champlain Center for Natural Medicine in Shelburne, Vermont.

Robert J. Zieve, M.D. is an author, lecturer, and practitioner of Integrative Biological Medicine. His practice includes homeopathy, European biological medicine, anthroposophical medicine, and nutrition. Dr. Zieve was medical director at Foxhollow Clinic in Louisville, Kentucky for two years and has a private practice in Louisville and in Chadford, Pennsylvania.

Part IV

Resources

➷ National Vaccine Information Center Questions

The National Vaccine Information Center (NVIC) recommends asking the following questions before vaccination:

1. Is my child sick right now?
2. Has my child had a bad reaction to a vaccination before?
3. Does my child have a personal family history of vaccine reactions, convulsions or neurological disorders, severe allergies or immune system disorders?
4. Do I know if my child is at high risk of reaction?
5. Do I have full information on the vaccine's side effects?
6. Do I know how to identify a vaccine reaction?
7. Do I know how to report a vaccine reaction?
8. Do I know the vaccine manufacturer's name and lot number?

For more information, contact:
National Vaccine Information Center
421-E Church Street
Vienna, VA 22180
(703) 938-0342
www.909shot.com

☞ Vaccine Information Resources

National Health Federation
P.O. Box 688
Monrovia, CA 91016
An immunization kit is available from the National Health Federation.

Vaccine Information and Awareness (VIA)
VIA produces an immunization/vaccine information package that will help you determine what is right for you and your child regarding vaccinations. If you have questions, call anyone on the resource lists or question your physician, health care practitioner, the manufacturer, the public health department, etc. Read, investigate, research, and question as much as you can until you feel you are fully informed about the vaccination decision.

The VIA packet, consolidated onto a floppy disk, contains:
- Article on freedom of choice vs. mandatory vaccinations
- Informed consent information sheet
- Patient bill of rights
- Resource list of pro-choice/information groups

- List of over seventy-five vaccine-related books and publications
- Comprehensive list of resources
- Package inserts from vaccine manufacturers
- Article on how to start a grassroots organization
- List of states who have a philosophical exemption
- Your individual state statute
- Religious exemption sample letter
- Current articles on vaccines

To obtain this information, visit the VIA website (home.san.rr.com/via) or contact:

Karin Schumacher, President and Founder
Vaccine Information and Awareness
12799 La Tortola
San Diego, CA 92129
(858) 454-3197
kschumacher@san.rr.com

Other sources of information about vaccines include:
- CDC, National Immunization Program:
  www.cdc.gov/nip
- National Vaccine Injury Compensation Program:
  www.hrsa.gov/osp/vicp
- Vaccine Adverse Event Reporting System, VAERS:
  www.fda.gov/cber/vaers/vaers.htm
- National Vaccine Information Center (NVIC):
  www.909shot.com

- "A Consumer's Guide to Vaccines," published by the National Vaccine Information Center, available by calling (800) 909-SHOT

Mailing Lists
To stay updated on the latest news you can join various vaccine lists. There's lots of support for parents who are still learning and trying to find a comfortable decision.

- Parents Requesting Open Vaccine Education (PROVE) (E-mail list)
  Go to www.vaccineinfo.net and select "Subscribe to PROVE Email News" to register.

- Adverse Vaccine Mailing List (AVML) (E-Mail List)
  Send an email to avml@topica.com. In the message body, type "Subscribe" and leave the subject line blank.

- The Australian Vaccination Network, Inc. (AVN) (E-Mail List)
  Go to www.onelist.com/subscribe.cgi/AVN for step-by-step instructions on how to subscribe, or send an empty email to AVN-subscribe@onelist.com.

- Parents talking to parents about medical issues
  Go to rainforest.parentsplace.com/dialog/get/vaccines3.html.

❧ Natural Medicine Resources

❧ Associations

National Center for Homeopathy
801 North Fairfax Street, Suite 306
Alexandria, VA 22314
www.homeopathic.org
Listings of practitioners, publications, workshops, and conferences.

Physicians Association for Anthroposophical Medicine (PAAM)
1923 Geddes Avenue
Ann Arbor, MI 48104
(734) 930-9462
www.paam.net
paam@anthroposophy.org
Names and addresses, conferences.

Anthroposophical Nurses Association of America (ANAA)

1923 Geddes Avenue

Ann Arbor, MI 48104

(734) 994-8303

www.artemisia.net/anaa

Anthroposophical nursing extends the traditional art and science of nursing to reflect a more complete picture of the developing human being. Anthroposphical nurses recognize the human being as a spiritual being in a human body. They walk with patients on their unique journey toward healing and know that the healing process ultimately rests within each individual. A course of study for registered nurses is available.

Association of Therapeutic Eurythmists in North America (ATHENA)

c/o Anne Cook

1081 Dickens Drive

Santa Rosa, CA 954017

(707) 568-4288

www.artemisia.net/athena

Eurythmy is an art of movement that brings the inner dynamics of speech and music to expression through movement and gesture. Its branch, therapeutic eurythmy, is an essential component of anthroposophically extended medicine. It allows the individual to actively participate in the prevention and treatment of illness. Therapeutic eurythmy is an uplifting and inspiring patient resource.

Rhythmical Massage Therapy Association

c/o Micky Leach

2501 West Zia Road

Santa Fe, NM 87505

(505) 438-0156

www.artemisia.net/rmta

Understanding that rhythm brings healing, this massage was developed in the 1920s by Dr. Ita Wegman who refined elaborate qualities of touch, enhancing the forces of lightness and levity through lifting and suction. At times when the pressures of life and illness weigh people down, the rhythmic, delicate quality of this form of treatment, is a great help.

Association for Anthroposophical Art Therapy in North America (AAATNA)

c/o Phoebe Alexander

437 East 80th Street, Apt. 5

New York, NY 10021

(212) 744-0257

phoenixartsgroup.org/aaatna

artopathy@aol.com

Goethe describes color as movement and activity arising where light and darkness meet. Light and darkness are reflections of the human being—the light of the ego meeting the darkness of substance. In diagnostic drawing and painting, done in a supportive setting, light, darkness, and color become outer representations revealing inner movement, and can be an important part of healing.

Anthroposophical Music Therapy

The task of music as healer is to rekindle the memory of the tonal world from which we all were formed. In learning to listen actively and to create sounds, the patient is led into his or her own deeper being. For this the lyre, a stringed instrument, is ideally suited. With simple exercises the music therapist creates a healing atmosphere, gradually fulfilling the silent longing to be in harmony with one's body and with the world.

For more information, contact:
Channa Seidenberg
(518) 672-4389

Creative Speech

A pioneering approach that accesses the health-giving, revitalizing forces inherent in the spoken word.

For more information, contact:
Judith Pownal
(312) 565-2477

Anthroposophical Society

General resource information. (734) 662-9355.

Camphill Association of America

For individuals in need of special care. (610) 469-6162.

❧ Natural Health Companies

Weleda Inc
175 Route 9W North
Congers, NY 10920
(800) 241-1030
www.weleda.com

Raphael Pharmacy
4003 Bridge Street
Fair Oaks, CA 95628
(800) 677-0015

American Association of Homeopathic Pharmacists
3741 Mitford Lane
Clinton, WA 98236
(800) 478-0421

Celletech
Started in England, Celletech carries forward the craft and tradition of producing high efficacy and quality homeotherapeutic products. For more detailed information, refer to www.celletech.com.

❧ Products

Peat Health Products
In the 1920s, Rudolf Steiner encouraged research in the development of clothing made from peat fibers. He indicated that at the end of the century it would be needed to protect human

beings against increased pollution and radiation. Peat, in the various therapeutic forms, offers the possibility of protection from the effects of radiation from energy devices, such as radio, TV, high-tension lines, computers, and nuclear power plants. Peat fibers gleaned from the upland moors of Sweden now serve as the basis for a variety of clothing articles, bedding, bath emulsions, massage oils and computer shields.

Peat has the following healing properties:
- Protects from undue outer influences.
- Has a warming and vitalizing effect.
- Soothes complaints due to sensitivity to weather changes.
- Helps bind and neutralize the products of body elimination (perspiration, odors, salts).
- Has natural bacteria-inhibiting properties.

For more information, contact:
Alyssa Canann
356 Ramona Way
Costa Mesa, CA 92627
(949) 645-7338

For product information, go to www.fortheloveofpeat.com or www.lachildhood.org.

Homecare Essentials
The purpose of Homecare Essentials is to expand the use of home remedies and practices to all who are drawn to them. Homecare supplies are made of natural fibers and are designed to treat common ailments at home. Each homecare kit contains wool, silk, and cotton wraps, compresses, and poultices; instruc-

tions; and a sample of organically grown chamomile tea. All are conveniently packaged in a kit to assist you in treating family members suffering from fevers, colds, and common ailments that can be treated at home.

For more information contact:
Mary Carmichael
12525 Parish Road
San Diego, CA 92128
(858) 673-5975

For product information, go to www.lachildhood.org.

Warmth as Healer
Lilling Company
P.O. Box 3571
Vero Beach, FL 32964
Toll-free: (800) 747-WOOL
Fax: (561) 234-6963
Cover brand: undyed merion wool soakers from Finland

Morning Rose
(877) 686-8200
www.childrenswoolens.com

Sierra Trading Post
sierratradingpost.com

❧ Recommended Reading

❧ Anthroposophical Literature

Practical Home Care Medicine: A Natural Approach, Christine Murphy, editor, Lantern Books, 2001

A Guide to Child Health, Wolfgang Goebel and Michaela Gloeckler, Anthroposophic Press, new edition due out January 2003

The Anthroposophical Approach to Medicine Vol. I, II, III, Husemann/Wolff, Anthroposophic Press, 1987

Spiritual Science and Medicine, Rudolf Steiner, Garber Communications, Inc., 1989

Anthroposophical Medicine, Dr. Michael Evans and Lain Rodger, Thorsons, 1992

Blessed by Illness, L. F. C. Mees, M.D., Anthroposophic Press, 1990

Living with your Body, Walther Buehler, Rudolf Steiner Press, 1979

Spiritual Science and the Art of Healing, Victor Bott, M.D., Healing Arts Press, 1996

Caring for the Sick at Home, T. van Bentheim, S. Bos, W. Visser, E. de la Houssaye, Floris Books/Anthroposophic Press, 1980

"The Art of Taking Care of a Sick Child," Miranda Castro, *Homeopathy Today,* a publication of the National Center for Homeopathy, February 2002

Further titles can be ordered from Steiner Books (Anthroposophic Press). See Publishing Companies, below.

❧ NVIC's Top Ten Vaccine Information Resources

1. *DPT: A Shot in the Dark,* Harris L. Coulter and Barbara Loe Fisher, Harcourt Brace Jovanovich, 1985; Warner Books, 1986; Avery, 1991; Penguin Putnam, 2000
   The book that launched the vaccine safety movement in America. Available as *A Shot in the Dark* in bookstores or from NVIC.

2. *The Consumer's Guide To Childhood Vaccines,* Barbara Loe Fisher, NVIC, 1997
   Short, concise guide to the risks and complications of ten childhood diseases and vaccines with glossary of medical terms.

3. NVIC website (www.909shot.com)
   This award-winning website is the oldest and largest consumer advocacy vaccine information website. Links to other vaccine information sources, from government health agencies to other consumer advocacy sources.

4. *What Your Doctor May Not Tell You About Children's Vaccinations*, Stephanie Cave, M.D., Warner Books, 2001
   A new, well-researched book that takes a closer look at current vaccine policies. Available from bookstores.

5. *DPT Vaccine And Chronic Nervous System Dysfunction (1994)*
   Adverse Events Associated With Childhood Vaccines (1994)
   Adverse Effects Of Pertussis And Rubella Vaccines (1991)
   Institute of Medicine reports published by National Academy Press in 1991 and 1994 after IOM-appointed physician committees reviewed the medical literature for evidence that vaccines can cause acute and chronic brain and immune system dysfunction. Copies of all three reports are available in limited quantities from the Division of Health Promotion and Disease Prevention, Institute of Medicine, 2101 Constitution Avenue, N.W., Washington, D.C. 20418.

6. *The Vaccine Guide*, Randall Neustaedter, OMD, North Atlantic Books, 1996

7. *What Every Parent Should Know About Childhood Immunizations*, Jamie Murphy, Earth Healing Products, 1993

8. "Vaccine Controversies," a special 32-page report in the August 26, 2000 issue of *The CQ Researcher* (Volume 10, No. 28, pp. 641-672). Published by Congressional Quarterly, Inc. For copies, call (800) 638-1710 or try your local library.

9. PROVE website (www.vaccineinfo.net)
Official website of Texas based consumer advocacy organization, PROVE (Parents Requesting Open Vaccine Education).

10. *Vaccines: Are They Really Safe And Effective?*, Neil Z. Miller, New Atlantean Press, 1992, 1999

➤ Publishing Companies

Steiner Books (Anthroposophic Press)
P.O. Box 960
Herndon, VA 20172
(800) 856-8664

Mercury Press
241 Hungry Hollow Road
Chestnut Ridge, NY 10977
(845) 425-9357

New Atlantean Press
(505) 983-1856
thinktwice.com/global.htm

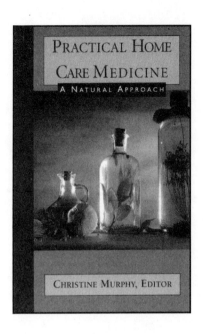

Simple treatments for many of the illnesses discussed in this book can be found in *Practical Home Care Medicine*, edited by Christine Murphy. Compiled from the notes and experiences of anthroposophical physicians, nurses, and patients, *Practical Home Care Medicine* lists some of their most frequently used non-prescription medicines, herb teas and kitchen remedies, and procedures. Use this book to enhance your partnership and collaboration with your physician, and to support your ingenuity and courage as a healer in your own home.